Practical social work

Published in conjunction with
the British Association of Social Workers
Series Editor: Jo Campling

B A S W

Social work is at an important stage in its development. The profession is facing fresh challenges to work flexibly in fast-changing social and organisational environments. New requirements for training are also demanding a more critical and reflective, as well as more highly skilled, approach to practice.

The British Association of Social Workers has always been conscious of its role in setting guidelines for practice and in seeking to raise professional standards. The concept of the *Practical Social Work* series was conceived to fulfil a genuine professional need for a carefully planned, coherent series of texts that would stimulate and inform debate, thereby contributing to the development of practitioners' skills and professionalism.

Newly relaunched, the series continues to address the needs of all those who are looking to deepen and refresh their understanding and skills. It is designed for students and busy professionals alike. Each book marries practice issues and challenges with the latest theory and research in a compact and applied format. The authors represent a wide variety of experience both as educators and practitioners. Taken together, the books set a standard in their clarity, relevance and rigour.

A list of new and best-selling titles in this series follows overleaf. A comprehensive list of titles available in the series, and further details about individual books, can be found online at :
www.palgrave.com/socialworkpolicy/basw/

Series standing order **ISBN 0–333–80313–2**

You can receive future titles in this series as they are published by placing a standing order. Please contact your bookseller or, in the case of difficulty, contact us at the address below with your name and address, the title of the series and the ISBN quoted above.

Customer Services Department, Macmillan Distribution Ltd, Houndmills, Basingstoke, Hampshire RG21 6XS, England

Practical social work series

New and best-selling titles

veronica coulshed and
audrey mullender

with

david n. jones and neil thompson

management in
social work

third edition

palgrave
macmillan

First edition 1990
Reprinted six times
Second edition 2001
Reprinted five times
Third edition 2006

Published by
PALGRAVE MACMILLAN
Houndmills, Basingstoke, Hampshire RG21 6XS and
175 Fifth Avenue, New York, N.Y. 10010
Companies and representatives throughout the world

PALGRAVE MACMILLAN is the global academic imprint of the
Palgrave Macmillan division of St. Martin's Press, LLC and of Palgrave
Macmillan Ltd. Macmillan® is a registered trademark in the United States,
United Kingdom and other countries. Palgrave is a registered trademark
in the European Union and other countries.

ISBN-13: 978–1–4039–1837–6
ISBN-10: 1–4039–1837–6

This book is printed on paper suitable for recycling and made from
fully managed and sustained forest sources. Logging, pulping and
manufacturing processes are expected to conform to the environmental
regulations of the country of origin.

A catalogue record for this book is available from the
British Library.

A catalog record for this book is available from the Library of Congress.

10   9   8   7   6   5   4   3
15   14   13   12   11   10   09   08

Printed in Great Britain by Creative Print & Design (Wales). Blaina

In memory of Veronica Coulshed

Contents

List of figures

Acknowledgement

The authors and publishers acknowledge with thanks permission from the President and Fellows of Harvard College to reproduce Figure 4.2, from R. Tannenbaum and W. H. Schmidt, 'How to choose a leadership pattern', *Harvard Business Review* (May–June 1973) © 1973 by the President and Fellows of Harvard College. All rights reserved.

Introduction

Since it was first published in 1990, this book has made an immeasurable contribution to the understanding and practice of management in social work. The second edition came out as the management and performance revolution was beginning to take hold in social service agencies, whilst our work on this third edition has taken place against a competing background of a continuing central government 'modernisation' agenda, on the one hand, and the tackling of complexity by postmodernist theory, on the other. Expanding the editorial team for this third edition, we retain the same commitment to improving standards as was evident in Veronica Coulshed's original text and continue to share her firm belief that good management plays a crucial role in achieving such progress.

Aims of the book

In writing this text, only shortly before her untimely death, Veronica Coulshed drew upon her whole career as a social worker, a team leader in a hospital and in social services, and a manager in social work education. This range of experiences had exposed her to the turmoil of cutbacks, uncertain futures and increasing demands. She was conscious of writing at a time when everyone in the human services – teaching, nursing and social work, for example – was being faced with the expectation that what they offered should become more efficient and effective. Living up to these requirements, she said, had underlined the need for everyone to manage and organise their work within administrative processes and managerial diktats which were sometimes made to feel more important than the people who operated them. Then, as now, social workers often tended to feel powerless at work. Some even scoffed at her notion that part of their role might be to learn how to question procedures, shape policy or improve services.

Veronica Coulshed was concerned by this alienation of staff, a concern that was belatedly accepted in the new millennium as the recruitment and retention of staff became a major political and managerial preoccupation. She wrote her book in the hope of lessening disillusionment with organisation and management, believing that to study these concepts would be to gain power through information. She further considered that learning about the influence of the context in which practice takes place would help social workers analyse their own performance at work.

Her central idea here, developed in Chapter 1, was that all social workers are managers. Their circles of activity ripple outwards from managing themselves, at the core, to managing others, and onwards again to managing systems. This concentration on managing oneself and other people is underpinned by theories about the nature of organisations and how they are structured. Working from the premise that frontline practitioners and managers can benefit from understanding these ideas, her book sought to translate a complex literature into workable, everyday knowledge. It also wrestled with making that literature more relevant to management in social work and to a human, as opposed to an abstract mechanistic, context. The hope was that, rather than feeling propelled by their agencies, readers might then be equipped to help change them.

Veronica Coulshed was concerned, too, that typical career pathways led many social workers out of direct practice and 'in at the deep end' of supervising others or managing teams. She recognised that too many employers failed to offer appropriate preparation or training for this change of role (still too often the case; McKay, 2002) and wanted, through her writing, to assist those who were moving into first line management positions by outlining the duties confronting them and exploring some of the skills and values which would help them become good managers. This third edition of her book again seeks to address those newly appointed and aspiring managers who wish to use their power responsibly and ethically, within a broader anti-oppressive agenda, for the promotion of social welfare and social justice.

Finally, but no less importantly, Veronica Coulshed hoped that the material she offered would be useful to students on qualifying programmes and she wanted everyone engaged in social work teaching and learning, as much as in social work practice and management, to acquire a critical stance towards their own endeavours. The National Occupational Standards for Social Work, in Key Role 5, call on the newly qualified social worker to demonstrate the ability to 'manage and be accountable, with supervision and support, for your own social work practice within your organisation' (see www.doh.gov.uk/swqualification/newrequirements.htm#app1). This encompasses a requirement to:

- Manage and be accountable for your own work
- Contribute to the management of resources and services
- Manage, present and share records and reports
- Work within multidisciplinary and multi-organisational teams, networks and systems.

The work-based learning approach of much of post-qualifying training in social work shares these objectives (even though there is an academic award under changes made by the General Social Care Council), so that the whole continuum of professional development for social workers has, in a sense, caught up with where Veronica Coulshed was well over a decade ago.

In working on this third edition, and from our combined almost ninety years' experience of social work practice, management and education, we, too, share this commitment to broadening educational concerns to encompass organisational issues, believing that social workers can empower others only if they feel as empowered as possible themselves within their employing agencies.

The managerial context of social work

Social workers have always been interested in being effective and making a difference, although many reacted against the dominant managerialism of the 1990s (see Clarke and Newman, 1997). In common with professionals in most other disciplines and human services, social work practitioners tend to hold negative attitudes towards the administrative and managerial aspects of their organisations and of their own workloads, often arguing that these are distractions from 'the real work'. Yet the time-consuming requirement to record assessments and care plans on computer, attend meetings, balance budgets and so on brings administration into the heart of social work and is an essential form of accountability to users and funders that cannot be avoided. The possibility has long gone of fieldworkers immersing themselves in their own self-contained activities and leaving administration to 'them' at county hall, the town hall or at headquarters (if they happen to work for a voluntary organisation).

All public services, including those services purchased by local councils from private or voluntary sector providers, must now demonstrate effectiveness and good value as part of their accountability to, and contract of trust with, the public. Although this involvement in management and service evaluation puts social workers in closer touch with what might be the creative potential of informing and influencing the translation of management information into policy development, in many places it has actually been experienced as a decisive shift to work that is routinised, rule-bound and more closely controlled by management. At one time it was possible for social workers in social services departments (SSDs), as 'street-level bureaucrats' (Lipsky, 1980), to function with a fair degree of discretion. Ironically, as the responsibilities of social workers have mushroomed, their autonomy seems correspondingly to have shrunk. Those who frame the policies designed to ration inadequate resources in the face of growing demand, or who feel exposed to public scrutiny if things go wrong, have been anxious to maintain a firm hold on all levels of decision-making so as to avoid legal challenge, official wrist-slapping or public criticism. Although government has stated principles of public sector improvement that involve greater delegation of authority to frontline staff, this time within clear national frameworks and standards, backed up by more discretion and improved pay (Blair, 2001), it is not yet clear that these aims will be realised in practice.

The 1980s saw an emphasis on the need for everyone in what the USA baptised the 'human service industry' to be efficient, effective and economical (the 'three Es'). No one would want to dispute the requirement to provide value for money when dispersing restricted public funds to a public with rising expectations, but, when market values and business criteria entered social work, some agencies did appear to forgo high standards of caring and safety in favour of enforcing the lowest cost. Nor was this only an in-house phenomenon in the statutory sector. Funding and grant requirements, set within the context of government policy, drove voluntary organisations, large and small, as well as newer private bodies, to trim costs and revise service levels. Local government services were increasingly contracted out to private sector (that is, profit-making) providers, while the voluntary sector employed marketing and business consultants, both to compete in this new market and raise funds from other sources. These moves towards a business ethos may well have deepened the already growing rift between social work professionals and their managers, with the two cultures apparently pursuing different ends.

Although considerations of cost are now unavoidable, low cost is not an absolute good. The notion of 'virtuous management' may sound like a contradiction in terms to those whose only experience has been of oppressive managerial cultures, but it does offer at least the potential that the discontinuity of values on becoming a manager, whether in the statutory, voluntary or private sector, is not preordained. For example, it is not essential to abandon an interest in service users on assuming supervisory control. One of this book's fundamental aims is to explore the links between social work and managerial approaches and values, that is, for combining the 'three Es' with compassion, integrity, and a determination to uphold the humane purposes of social welfare organisations. Since the publication of the first edition, it has been good to see something of a resurgence of interest in public service values as underpinning good management (Steele, 1999; Jones, 2000).

This may all sound somewhat obvious to those managers who are naturally good at steering a course through conflicting philosophies. But a reading of management literature will quickly illustrate that, until recently, some rather devious and even brutal qualities of leadership have been not only admired but recommended. This book will re-examine such thinking from the perspective of those who reject the image of the ruthless, single-minded manager who is wily about office politics and who can get the better of subordinates, competitors and superiors alike – the manager who thinks that all problems can be solved by the mechanical use of rational-technical tools, such as flow charts, procedural manuals and decision-making models.

It is a pleasure to report that management theory has itself been moving away from such gamesmanship towards what is known as the 'feminisation' of management styles. Both male and female managers are being encouraged to value networking and cooperative decision-making over lone, competitive point-scoring because the organisation stands to gain most when all its best minds are on board and when all are free to contribute their own ideas, however greatly these diverge from the traditional 'norm'.

Veronica Coulshed was characteristically ahead of her time in writing about women colleagues in social work trying to persuade their managers to see that concern for people at work and honest relationships were signs of strength, not weakness. She appreciated the full irony of business and industry catching onto these ideas – the traditional territory of social work practice, one might have thought – just at the time when social work managers were belatedly adopting the traditional 'masculine' approaches of leading from the centre in leaner and fitter organisations that devalue and discard those who fail to toe the line or those squeezed out by reorganisation and 'downsizing'. While financial corporations were valuing the contribution of women by starting to provide crèche facilities and flexible working arrangements, while design firms were sharing power in 'flat' hierarchies where everyone sat round one large table and pooled creative ideas, while industry was introducing 'quality circles' where workers at all levels shared the input into management ideas, and while businesses of all kinds advertised for leaders with good communication and interpersonal skills, an open style and accessible manner, social work management was abandoning the profession's roots in just these individual and group-based skills. Company directors were being urged to 'become obsessed with listening', 'defer to the front line' and 'practise visible management' (Peters, 1988) at a time when social service and probation managers were centralising control away from area or district teams and imposing ever more rigid ordering and controlling on the work of staff they rarely met.

It is not difficult to understand why this might be. Social work operates under the pressure of legislation, political control, policy imperatives, media attention, and numerous other influences beyond the strictly professional. New Labour, with its centralising modernisation agenda, has responded to revelations of sexual abuse in residential settings and poor management in some authorities with aggressive talk of regulating and controlling social work activity, training and entry into the profession. There is a political search for 'core functions' and unequivocal statements about the need to base practice on clear evidence of 'what works'.

Yet we return to Veronica Coulshed's advice that the existence of so few 'certainties' on becoming a manager might mean that the occupation of social work would be best served by admitting to service users and the wider public that it does not have all the answers and that there are limitations to its resources, human and otherwise. Whatever management technologies may have to offer – and they are certainly an improvement on autocratic whim – there remains a need to stress to all social work's stakeholders that many aspects of the work rest on uncertainty and unpredictability, and that, despite published procedures, risk assessments, computerisation and workload review systems, some mistakes will continue be made. There may be firm high ground where we can make ready use of management theory and skills, but those familiar with Schön's (1983) ideas on 'reflective practice' will recognise the 'swampy lowlands' of human distress where professional decision-making is far more complex than the current obsession with occupational standards and competences would suggest (Ixer, 1999). This book will aim to face up to daily life as it really is for social workers and to look at management theory from their vantage point, in the belief that it does contain much material that is quite – and some that is very – useful to the busy practitioner or team leader.

The central problem with a faith in narrowly defined, 'top-down' managerial competence, underpinned by administrative good order and rationality, is that it is simply incapable of sorting out the untidiness of human difficulties or the uncertainties of direct practice in social work or social care. Social work organisations exist to serve messy, untidy, infinitely varied human beings and, indeed, all organisations are (at least up to now) staffed by them. Even were this not the case, so much is expected of managers today that it would probably be impossible to live up to the promises held out to the public by the issuing of neat lists of eligibility thresholds, service priorities or performance indicators, let alone the prescriptions of some of the earliest thinkers on management technique that we will encounter in the historical pages of this book. It is useful, then, to see a newer generation of theory arising, linking management studies and work in the public services, including social work, in a less output-driven understanding that allows for far greater complexity (Haynes, 2003). The recognition that constant change requires more flexible thinking by managers and more adaptable structures in organisations may cast into doubt how predictable and orderly the world can be, but it leaves plenty of scope for the creativity and people skills in which social work has always excelled.

A note on terminology and language

A note about terms which might be confusing or misunderstood may be helpful at this point. First, while being fully aware of subtle differences between them, Veronica Coulshed used the terms 'manager', 'administrator' and 'leader' interchangeably in order to avoid repetition. She also did so to emphasise her view that all social workers are managers, in the sense that 'management' can be defined as the process of organising resources to get work done. At the same time, she recognised that the management of people is a far more varied business than dealing with policies on paper, and she pointed to Warham's (1975) analysis of administration as a generic process in which direction, management and supervision are key elements. In this formulation, if 'administration' refers to the over-all process, then the component elements correspond to three general levels in the hierarchy: at the top, the directing function involves long-term planning and objectives; in the middle, the management function sustains the system as a going concern; while the supervisory function at the team leader level oversees the use of the resources and policy instructions provided by management to ensure that performance is up to standard. In a small private or voluntary agency, the directing, managing and supervising functions may be vested in one person, but more usually they are divided up.

Next, the term 'bureaucracy' is used here as a neutral concept which denotes a particular facet of organisational structure, not in the disparaging usage common in social work. As will be shown in Chapter 2, the concept did not have any pejorative connotation originally, but can be used as a yardstick of formality and imper-sonality in any organisation. Similarly, 'professionalism' is used in the positive sense of implying proficiency, an appropriate mainte-nance of personal and professional boundaries and a commitment to high standards; while 'professionalisation' signifies only a process of developing towards an 'ideal' type of model for the organisation of a particular form of work (with registration with the General Social Care Council marking another step along the way), and does not carry any connotation of being preoccupied with power or status.

Although the profession has seen a fragmentation into new organisational configurations and new roles, and although government sees 'social care' as a wider term, we shall continue to use the term 'social work' as the generic one. It remains the designation that is globally understood to encompass both the profession and the academic discipline with which we are concerned here and we retain our pride in it as encompassing a shared concern for social welfare, social justice and social action.

We have the usual annoying English habit of writing about 'social services' and 'local authorities' as if these terms covered the organisation of social work and social care in the statutory sector throughout the UK. We are well aware that Scotland has social work services and that Northern Ireland's equivalent provision is run by Trusts. We also use the term to cover both adult and children's services, even where formally divided but confess that we find it difficult to maintain a flow while also naming these alternatives.

Other aspects of language may have changed since this book first appeared. The talk in many settings now is of 'service users' or 'customers' rather than 'clients', for example, and new coinages appear all the time, such as 'benchmarking' and 'hot desking'. Throughout the text, we have attempted to use expressions that are currently the most widely used or recognisable, rather than necessarily closest to Veronica Coulshed's original.

Producing this edition

In one other, critically important way, revising this book has not presented any problem of language whatsoever. When Audrey Mullender and Veronica Coulshed first met, they felt as if they already knew each other from reading each other's work. They felt an affinity, particularly, in the fact that each had seen in the other's output an effort always to write in plain English, no matter how complicated the idea being discussed. They felt this was something they had in common and that it was likely to mean they would get on. They were right, although sadly they had little time to get to know one another before Veronica's untimely death.

This commitment to communicate clearly in all that Veronica wrote – her drive to reach the widest audience with the fewest possible obstacles – has made it a positive pleasure to work on this text. There has never been the slightest doubt what Veronica was driving at or what personal and professional commitment lay behind her commentary on the issue in question. Veronica was a natural communicator and teacher, someone about whom generations of students continue to say that she helps them understand things they have really struggled with until coming across her work. Veronica's ability to summarise without oversimplifying, her choice of only the most useful references and her knack with helpful illustrations all add to the 'readability' of her book and have all been retained in essence in this edition. That is not to say that the revised text stays especially close to the original. So much has moved on, and so quickly, that it has felt truer to what Veronica herself would have done to grasp the nettle of major change in the hope of ensuring that no reader's interest or understanding is lost along the way. As a result, although all four of our names appear on the spine, we three who came later must accept the lion's share of blame for any infelicities or inaccuracies in this revised edition.

That said, we want to pay tribute to Veronica for being so far ahead of her time in spotting many of the 'coming' trends. The purchaser–provider split, the introduction of a new managerialist ethos and the countervailing trend elsewhere towards a broadening of what counts as good management were all, for example, firmly located in her text a decade and a half ago and they remain equally important now. But no one, not even she, could have foreseen the pace of change in social work throughout the 1990s and into the new millennium.

Structure of the book

The book begins by proposing in Chapter 1 that we are all managers and emphasising, therefore, why it is useful for social work staff at whatever level to study management ideas. Chapter 2 sketches in the background of thinking about organisational structures and theories about management and people at work. The rise in the requirement to demonstrate that users are receiving the best possible services is reflected in a new focus for Chapter 3 around models of quality standards and the management of change, with a role envisaged for all staff in helping to move things forward. In Chapter 4, the focus shifts to the designated leaders of social work organisations and their key contribution in terms of managerial vision and strategic planning. Chapters 5 and 6 consider the human resource side of management, that is, the recognition that a welfare organisation's biggest investment is in its staff. This means that it cannot hope to operate effectively unless it puts in place good policies and practices on all staffing matters, starting from recruitment and selection and progressing through integrated systems for staff appraisal, staff development and staff care. Since there can be no quality without equality, diversity is the focus of Chapter 7.

Having laid out all the responsibilities that managers carry in today's social work agencies, finally, in Chapter 8, we examine what scope there may be for individual managers to find their own styles and to empower others to give of their best, as opposed to abusing the power inherent in organisational leadership under the guise of 'running a tight ship'. Management (although not managerialism) could, it is argued, actually liberate social work to pursue not only its early values of respect for persons, but also new principles of equality, social justice and the highest achievable standards of service for hitherto marginalised and devalued groups within society.

Audrey Mullender, with David Jones
and Neil Thompson

1 | Why study management?

This chapter outlines why it is useful for social workers at every level to know something of the discipline called 'management'. It asserts that all social workers are managers of a kind and debates whether, to look at this the other way round, all managers in social work organisations should have a background in social work practice. Regardless of one's views on this question, it does have to be accepted that today's managers employ not only many skills which are transferable from practice but also others peculiar to the management world, in scope if not always in detail.

The relevance of management theory to social work

As social work organisations move through an era of fragmentation, discontinuity, contracting out and delayering, each staff member is finding a need to understand how organisational systems work. This is essential both to survival and to finding one's own place in the scheme of things. It also makes sense among ever increasing managerial demands for detailed information and budgetary accountability. Every social worker is having to learn to think on a much broader canvas than has ever been the case before. This involves looking outwards to service users and resource providers – as well as to politicians who increasingly expect to set the agenda – looking back over work that needs to be monitored and reviewed, and forwards in order to plan and set aims and objectives. This breadth of vision is something that managers have always needed and the management literature has useful things to say on the subject.

Thinking like a manager also enables social workers to bring a critical eye to bear on their own organisations, the services they provide and the standards they set. When people are busy, they sometimes forget to stand back and reflect on how they are perceived, especially by users. Developing a dispassionate approach to what is going on is beneficial; a detached concern helps to maintain a questioning, analytical stance regarding how services are delivered and received. Each time we approach the reception desk of an area office, or visit a group care establishment, it is salutary to ponder on how we would feel if we were a service user or a resident there. There is nothing sadder than to visit an elderly relative or a former neighbour in a home and find that, despite good standards of physical care, their individuality is being eroded because staff are not encouraged to consider their own behaviour in relation to the organisation's primary objectives. This always reflects on the skills, abilities and motivation of the managers, who may be preoccupied with financial profit in the private sector, short-term cost control in the public sector or simply seeking a quiet life.

Through studying management, too, we can try to prevent ourselves becoming mere instruments of managerialism or its scapegoat if something goes wrong. Some employers, for instance, have not been beyond disowning the judgements of their staff, even when their own position in the hierarchy made them ultimately responsible for training and supporting those individuals. The relevance of management studies to social work might lie in helping us to see when it is the system, not ourselves, that is at fault and when standards are not good enough and need changing.

Why all social workers are managers

The suggestion that all social workers are managers is probably, at first glance, not a welcome one. Similarly, those who are about to become managers may be facing the transition with mixed feelings – while keen to learn the techniques and gain the rewards of the competent leader, they may also fear losing touch with direct practice and perhaps becoming deskilled. The stereotype of a manager is of a person (disproportionately likely to be male) who has sacrificed social work values to the importance of filling in forms or gathering data on computer and who gives priority to what his manager in turn expects rather than what users and practitioners demand. Yet, in fact, many practitioner skills in social work are also managerial ones, and all social workers increasingly work to managerialist agendas, so the difference may be one of degree rather than of kind. It has been exaggerated by practitioners not knowing what their managers really do and by a failure on both sides to appreciate that working to change an organisation is not so very far removed from the mainstay of social work itself.

The most obvious overlap concerns the management of people. Whether these be service users, carers, the general public or those who regulate service provision, management, just like practice, involves the ability to write and speak clearly and to engage in purposeful interpersonal relationships. So perhaps social workers who become managers have a head start here? On the other hand, believing that they 'should' have a flair for 'people skills' could embarrass those who are newly promoted, impeding spontaneity and making them self-conscious for a time. It may help to remember that managing people is at the heart both of providing services to users through social work methods and of organising and working towards the effective delivery of those services by others.

The principles and skills involved in managing personnel are common to all organisations – private, public and voluntary. The objectives may be different from one agency to another, and at each level within a department, but the means used in attempting to reach them remain constant. Engaging with and relating to people, helping others to achieve their goals, supervising their efforts, maintaining morale, consulting a wide range of sources prior to making decisions, problem-solving, and introducing and managing the process of change are just some of the tasks common to the practitioner and the manager.

There are also transferable skills from particular methods and modes of social work intervention. The systemic thinking which underlies the techniques of family therapy, for example, is just as relevant when trying to sort out the patterns of relationships which exist in larger systems such as organisations as it is in families. Equally, when leading a team, many of the ideas gleaned from groupwork also stand one in good stead. Just as Allan Brown (1992) proposes that those who have experienced mutually trusting, collaborative and creative teams make good groupworkers, so those with experience of groupwork are likely to contribute to positive team spirit and constructive co-working as facilitative team members or team leaders. Knowledge of group cohesion, openness, risk-taking and interdependence in groups can be transferred directly to the role of team manager, although the context and aims naturally differ from those experienced in groupwork intervention.

A further good preparation for management is the role of the care manager. Undertaking assessments and coordinating packages of care within tight budgets has become a core task for many front-line practitioners. Valuable skills developed include those of bargaining, mediating, negotiating, liaising and advocacy in order to make the best use of resources. And one could certainly argue that social workers who have become more financially aware, even without holding the purse strings of a fully devolved budget, will make better managers later on. There will be less of a divide to cross than in the days before unit costs of service were known, when social workers were largely unaware of the direct impact of resource restraints and decisions to refuse services were taken much higher up the hierarchy than may be the case now.

For those social workers who are budget holders, there may be some worrying issues to be resolved. For instance, there may be inherent contradictions in orchestrating community care packages within resource limitations while also acting as an advocate for better client services overall, or in balancing a user's needs and wishes while also shopping around for the least costly forms of care. Although we may not argue with the need to keep the taxpayer in mind, there is the problem that, when professionals are given financial responsibility, they may become distracted from their fundamental aims. As Priestley (1998) demonstrates in respect of care assessments of disabled people, these frequently appear to be budget-led rather than truly needs-led, and the discourse of 'need' is in any case contentious since it usually covers only personal and domestic tasks, not assistance in having a social life, for example. It remains to be seen whether direct payment schemes will give service users more access to real choice and whether social workers will learn from disabled people that they do not have a monopoly on defining need.

Although these narrowly financial concerns may be recent, the management of resources has, in fact, always dominated the social worker's tasks if we count within this the management of time and of self. Frontline workers devote many hours to travelling, attending meetings, negotiating, doing 'admin' and referring on. It is startling how many social workers and their managers are unable to ration themselves across a working day or week or to delegate effectively. While the theme of the 1980s was to assume that managers should be available at all times and respect was reserved for the 'workaholics' (the 'lunch is for wimps' ethos), the managers of the future (and ideally all workers) should be noted for their capacity to reflect on what they are doing and to draw boundaries around the energies available for their career and those available for personal and family commitments. (Lunch is back in fashion, as is building exercise and 'quality time' into the day.) Self-management of this nature is one way of preventing stress-related illness.

As well as managing resources, social workers and social care staff at all levels participate in meeting required standards. In child care policy and practice, for example, individual social workers are told very clearly what information they need to gather about children and families in the Assessment Framework, the Looked After Children (LAC) Assessment and Action Records, and the national codes and guidelines for both foster care and the residential care of children. Standards for adult services, too, are enforced by independent scrutiny and all services are being drawn into National Service Frameworks to ensure effective working across professional and organisational boundaries.

Standards and procedures are equally a part of a new ethos in the voluntary and private sectors. Most voluntary organisations have to comply with Charity Commission requirements and often the obligations of a compact and/or contracts with the local authority, and all independent providers operate within a contract culture, which means that staff have to be constantly aware of quality standards and required managerial practices. Nor do freelancers escape from procedures, guidelines and form-filling. Trainers, consultants, mentors and other self-employed people who use their social work qualifications and experience to work from home are increasingly expected to operate their own quality controls to nationally recognised standards and the contracts they obtain for their services typically require this to be the case.

A final reason why we would argue that all social workers are managers is that each person in a department can be an instigator or a contributor to change and innovation. These do not always have to come from outside; changing the agency from within occurs quite frequently and one need not always be in a position of power to influence agency practice. If we view organisations as psycho-socio-political systems and study people's behaviour within them, we are then in a good position to change our working practices, especially if, in their current form, they are adding to the burdens of users, carers and others. Undertaking projects for Post Qualifying and Advanced Award programmes in social work or for an MBA is one opportunity that increasing numbers of people have had for standing back and thinking about a focused area of work where they can be particularly influential.

What is special about managers?

It may be that some readers will disagree with the assertion that social workers are practitioner-managers. It could fairly be pointed out that being a manager consists of more than undertaking managerially dictated duties; there are specific tasks involved, not least enabling others to get work done and carrying forward the overall aims of the organisation. So let us consider a few of the ways in which managers' functions are distinct.

First, while managers and social workers both control resources and exercise authority, the extent to which they do so differs. Second, the social worker is a specialist in delivering the services from her/his particular domain, whereas a manager's tasks relate to the organisation as a whole or at least one section of it. Thus, those who control group care services would take into account additional factors when deciding to allocate a place in an establishment to an older person, including the overall policy of the agency and the total number of people competing for the resource. Managers have to make decisions and be concerned for clients whom they have never met. Third, although practitioners keep an eye to the future when planning their work on a particular case, top managers have a macro-interest in the future of the whole organisation, ensuring that it will remain a going concern to meet future needs while also dealing with ever changing current circumstances. Fourth, social work and management processes share a concern for problem-solving and enabling, but the degree of authority in organising people to get work done is greater for line managers. In addition, styles of leadership and the performance of managerial tasks, such as the exercise of authority through decision-making, have an effect on other people's performance, not simply one's own; thus, the size of caseloads, the allocation of work and the supervision of it are usually part of the duties of team leaders and senior members of staff. Finally, the selection and orientation of new staff, although involving the team, is normally a specific task for people in management positions.

Before we move on to explore another side of this coin, by questioning if all managers should be social workers, let us recap the position so far:

1. Managerial administration is the process of *organising resources to get work done* and, at this level of generality, all social workers are involved in it.
2. Although certain roles carry the title of manager, team leader or senior, in every organisation each person is part of the administrative structure and is thus administratively, as well as professionally, *accountable for the work they do.*
3. At the same time, managers who have this title have specific functions that are *essential ingredients of their role as administrators*; some of these are different in degree rather than kind from the work of social workers, but others are related to the authority which is exercised.

Should all managers be social workers?

Is it necessary for those who develop and maintain social welfare organisations to be qualified social workers? When social services departments (SSDs) were first created, it was thought that those heading them should, if possible, be qualified in social work and, ideally, be experienced and/or trained in administration (Seebohm Report, 1968). At that time, many top managers were promoted through the practitioner ranks and only a few were from other professions. Management training and qualifications were poorly developed; experience and 'political' ability were seen as the key requirements. The rise of the managerial ethos in the 1990s undermined this position, with generic management training and skills coming to the fore. At the same time, SSDs themselves started to diversify and increasingly employed a variety of professionals, notably nurses and occupational therapists, to undertake roles in adult services. More recently, not only have social work-qualified managers started to disappear but also the social services as a separate entity. Various forms of restructuring have taken place. In England and Wales, children's social services are splitting away from adult services, with Children's Trusts now bringing children's social services and a range of other services for children and young people, such as health and education, together in one, new organisational structure. In some, Care Trusts perform a similar function for adult services. At the same time, social workers are increasingly employed outside these settings altogether, in multidisciplinary teams of various kinds. In all these examples, there is no reason why the team or organisational managers should be from a social work background.

In the voluntary sector, there are equally significant changes. Charitable organisations have had to become more businesslike, more competitive in an age of contracting out, are held to account for their performance and are reliant on marketing their image and their work in order to sustain an income; their managers face new challenges accordingly (Jackson and Donovan, 1999). Of course, there is enormous diversity among voluntary bodies in the UK and only a fraction have a social work identity or even employ qualified social workers, although, at the same time, there is a continuing trend for local authorities to contract out public services to voluntary sector provider agencies. The question of who their 'managers' should be is therefore complex. The private sector has also increasingly entered social care, as a provider of a wider range of services, bringing its own ethos of customer relations and financial management. It is not uncommon for managers to run their own care homes or be employed in relatively small businesses. A social work qualification would not be high on the list of requirements for such a position.

All these developments radically change the balance of the argument about what is needed in a manager. When even well established charities are having to look for figureheads who are good at 'fronting' their organisations, the idea of being professionally qualified in social work may seem almost irrelevant. And the emphasis on commercial or business 'success' may dictate a different set of priorities and skills from those traditionally valued by organisations which see themselves as preventing human distress and working in partnership with users – for whom there may be little public sympathy or support.

Moreover, just as good teachers or good nurses do not necessarily make good managers, experienced social workers may not make an automatic transition, either. The specific tasks of management administration outlined above, and the broader perspective that is required of social work leaders, are not part of everyone's equipment. If we look back to the Introduction, it was suggested that administration combines the three elements of *direction* (long-term planning), *management* (sustaining the system as a going concern) and *supervision*. If, as we said, these correspond with three general levels in the hierarchy, then we might be able to answer the question by proposing that, in large organisations, the two top tiers primarily call for sound management (and are precisely the levels at which staff are increasingly studying for MBAs), while the supervisory roles are best carried by those who have competence in the professional activity they are supervising. Interesting backing for this view comes from a study which shows that third-tier social service managers mainly do have professional qualifications, but that their thinking may well turn to obtaining management training once they begin to move up the career ladder; they begin to identify as managers rather than as social workers (Lawler and Hearn, 1997). Nevertheless, it is only in the most senior roles that professional managers are starting to be seen, that is, those who have trained in generic management skills and have chosen to use them in the public sector, as opposed to those who have risen through the ranks to a top-level management post.

The appointment of people with social work qualifications and backgrounds to key posts in Primary Care Trusts, combined local authority departments and other multidisciplinary settings demonstrates that social workers have a great deal to offer at all levels. Their experience in relating to other professionals and their organisations equips them well for managing multidisciplinary teams, and they benefit from the fact that both management and social work are all about people and relationships. It would be a shame if more social workers did not aim for the top, including women, black staff and others who have traditionally been under-represented at that level. Adding mentoring, management training and skills on the way up can only help. Whoever is given the role of manager, a solid grounding in the nature of the service being provided, credibility with staff and an understanding of the roles of those in direct contact with the public are essential.

Whatever the position held in a social work organisation, there are certain commitments that all managers have to make and particular challenges to address, as listed below:

1. Despite, and in some senses because of, the breadth of issues tackled in the personal social services, this is nevertheless a highly *specialised field.*

2. Social workers have their own *skills, knowledge and values.*
   As professionals, their expertise in planning and decision-
   making within their own field has to be acknowledged
   and mirrored in the way the agency involves them in
   administrative processes.
3. Any plans for developing services or rethinking the agency's
   mission (that is, its purpose) need to reflect the *equal
   opportunities goals* that have become part of social work's
   traditions, including a commitment to anti-oppressive
   practice.
4. If the manager comes from a different occupational
   background, credibility might be established more readily by
   showing a genuine willingness to learn about social work's
   current professional concerns and practices.
5. The importance of *relationships* needs to be highlighted:
   between service users and workers; among team members;
   with other disciplines; and also with numerous local, regional
   and national bodies.
6. What distinguishes human service management from that
   in non-service sectors is the fact that many agencies are
   dependent upon other organisations; planning has to take
   into account the *restraints* imposed by legislation and policy
   imposed from outside, as well as those inherent in relying on
   others to purchase or provide services.
7. Management approaches in social work cannot always be the
   rational and *tidy* ones suggested in some of the management
   literature. Service goals may contradict one another (for
   example caring versus controlling antisocial behaviour) and
   there are additional demands in making services holistic and
   appropriate rather than fragmented or impersonal, as well as
   in matching them wherever possible to the felt needs of a
   particular community (for instance in providing home care
   services which are acceptable to people of varying ethnic
   backgrounds).
8. Human services operate in *turbulent environments,* frequently
   subject to political whims and media-led changes, therefore
   long-term plans have to be flexible.
9. While coping with all this uncertainty, the manager of a
   service organisation also has to recognise that staff work
   from imperfect theories and conflicting ideologies about the

'causes' of human behaviour, they are called upon to tackle unpredictable and unknowable events and they increasingly focus largely on the 'heavy end' of human distress and need, as in child protection and mental health services. This makes *staff care* and *staff development* particularly important in social work, but also means that any requests from management are likely to be experienced as yet one more demand from those who are not actually involved in doing the frontline job.

10. Perhaps most importantly, the commitment of social work managers must not be to the organisation as an end in itself or to their own personal ambitions. The *raison d'être* of social work is its *service users and the general public more widely*; consequently, the focus has to be on high quality services and on supporting, developing, monitoring and guiding the work of the professionals who implement them.

The challenge to management outlined in this book is to harness management theories and those styles in social work which are best suited to the developments of the new millennium. The time is overdue to flush out managerial approaches which may have sounded impressive or 'macho' in their day but which have proven unable to balance the requirements of a principled and intelligent workforce, a vulnerable but potentially self-determining body of users and their carers and a general public which, while committed to the maintenance of high quality welfare services, also cares about community safety, good stewardship of public (or charitable) money and the public mandating of trends in social policy. If this makes management sound as if it is all about listening to, and working with, an infinite variety of people while undertaking a taxing job, then social workers ought to be extremely good at it! And, of course, many of them are.

2 | Management theory and organisational structures

In this chapter, we examine some of the best known approaches to management, the structure of organisations, and the thinking that both shapes people's behaviour and is shaped by it. Starting from the classical theories of management, we look at: scientific managerialism, which tends to treat employees like cogs in a machine; the human relations school of management theory which added people into the equation; and the study of organisational structures, particularly bureaucratic hierarchies and organisations as systems, because these models will be most familiar to social workers. (Later chapters will consider the culture of excellence, with its emphasis on quality, and other current trends, including reward management.)

Within each approach we explore the key contributions of some of the main pioneers associated with that school of thought. This is, after all, the world of management gurus and top business executives who sometimes become better known than the ideas they promote or the products they sell. A key source for the whole chapter will be Clutterbuck and Crainer (1990), who provide a fascinating account of the lives of these formative thinkers and doers (although their book is not geared towards the public sector).

The social workers of today will recognise throughout this chapter the competing trend towards maximising efficiency and recognising the contribution of people – the human resource – to the workplace. They will also find a number of ideas and terms they recognise but the origins of which may be less familiar.

It may seem odd in a book focusing on management in social work to look at ideas developed chiefly in the worlds of manufacturing and commerce. Nevertheless, just like workers on the factory floor or shop assistants, social workers are part of complex organisations – which can help or hinder them in delivering services. And, equally, the individual practitioner, or the area or district team, can be perceived by management as a help or a hindrance to achieving organisational goals. People's experiences of being in social work will be influenced, then, not only by their own efforts and abilities, but also by many other factors. These include: the shape of the organisation; the way the job is organised within it (including the degree of devolved control over decision-making and resource allocation); and the whole culture of the workplace. Increasingly, the demands on social work agencies are intensifying, not only to improve their own internal functioning but also to turn outwards to work in partnership with other agencies and be responsive to the expectations of the general public and particular user groups. No agency can just muddle through on acquired wisdom or good intentions. This is why social work managers are increasingly seeking MBA qualifications, S/NVQs in management (or their equivalent), Diplomas in Management Studies or other formal qualifications, and why social workers themselves need to have some understanding of how their agencies work at the organisational level. This chapter provides a useful starting point.

Scientific managerialism: classical theories

Henri Fayol: principles of management

Organisations do not manage themselves. If policy is to be uniformly followed and resources fairly allocated, communication and coordination have to be deliberately facilitated. The first rational approach to organising an enterprise was taken by Fayol (1841–1925), a French mining engineer who rose to become the managing director of the company that employed him. It was Fayol who defined management, in writings up to 1916, both in terms of its elements (what managers do) and its principles (how they can do it most effectively).

The means Fayol used to pull his company round from the brink of collapse are still familiar to us today in the form of: annual and 10-year business plans; organisational charts in which every post has its definite place; recruitment and training to ensure that the right person holds each post; top-down command and direction of the organisation; control of the whole enterprise on the basis of clear and rapidly prepared accounting data (which we would now broaden to 'management information'); and meetings of divisional and departmental heads, presided over by one manager who coordinates all their work. Fayol is probably best remembered for his 14 principles of management, among the most important of which for our purposes are the following:

1. *Those at the top are responsible for identifying key objectives.* We shall return to this, Fayol's 'unity of direction', under the fashionable label of 'mission statement', in Chapter 4.
2. *Specialisation is achieved by dividing groups to undertake similar functions.* In social work, this can be by user group, problem type, method of working, setting or context, population group, practice role, specific tasks, or stage in the allocation and progress of the work.
3. *Each worker should report to only one senior.* This, again, is a principle still followed today, although there can be complications with it, as we shall see below.
4. *Each person should have a job description.* This is ever more important – see Chapter 5.
5. *The ideal 'span of control'.* That is, it was thought that the number of people doing similar work supervised by one person should be six to eight. Senior social workers may end up supervising more than this, especially when covering vacant posts.

Critique and legacy of Fayol's ideas

Critiques of Fayol's work (see, for example, Drucker, 1977) point out that he based much of his theory, his 'functional principle', on a relatively small-scale company, employing one kind of worker to do one kind of job, with a single product (coal) which needed very little done to it before it could be sold, and serving only a few markets in which it had a virtual monopoly. He rested too much on this one example. His design principle is not well adapted to complexity, size, innovation or externally imposed change, all of which feature heavily in social work. He also assumed top-down management – forecasting and planning being, in Fayol's view, the main task of the organisational head – rather than the participation, partnership and teamwork of which there is so much talk today, or the answerability to outside interests, like government and the local community, that pertain in social work.

The key limitation in Fayol's thinking lay in trying to prescribe one set of principles to cover all eventualities. Yet, for some time, others continued in this line. Luther Gulick, for example, believed that any organisation could be as efficient as a piece of machinery if sound management practices were introduced, with both work and power divided according to an overall plan. As a result of analysing the executive tasks carried out by the US government in the 1930s, he coined the acronym PODSCORB – Planning, Organising, Directing, Staffing, Coordinating, Reporting, Budgeting. These functional elements of administration certainly have to be covered by any management structure, and Gulick's work still has influence, but it fell at the end of the period when management thinkers tried to devise simple, generalisable recipes for success.

Eventually, empirical research led by Joan Woodward in the 1950s revealed that there are, in fact, no optimum structural characteristics (such as number of levels of hierarchy or ideal span of control) or principles of administration that apply to all organisations. What affects success is the fit between structure, task, technology, management, employees and environment. These therefore came to be studied in a more holistic way in later work (see human relations and systems approaches, below).

Frederick W. Taylor: 'Scientific management'

Taylor (1856–1917) was the originator of the movement known as 'scientific management' or 'Taylorism': 'perhaps the first true management movement' (Clutterbuck and Crainer, 1990, p. 24). Just as Fayol tried to make management rational, Taylor tried to make specific tasks rational, drawing on his lifelong interests in engineering and inventing. He set about systematically studying work, breaking each task down into its component movements to discover the most efficient way of performing each job, and then considered how management techniques could control the workers to work consistently at maximum efficiency.

Everyone is familiar with his methods – the stopwatch and the 'time and motion' study – and with their outcomes in the form of piece-rate working and incentive schemes. He looked at people as if they were machines, except that humans make errors and, in his view, work only to earn money (albeit money that can buy a better quality of life outside work). Taylor's interest in management lay in not allowing people to make machines less efficient than they ultimately could be.

The worst excesses of this approach may have been tempered in the UK by the trade union movement, and more recently by a better understanding of what makes people tick, but its legacy lives on. Whenever we hear talk of output measures, functional analysis of occupations, performance indicators and so on, we are in the world of Taylorism. Care managers may also be interested to hear that, as a management consultant, Taylor introduced systematic purchasing and supply procedures, while his rigorous inspections of quality (with even the quality inspectors being audited) also has a familiar ring.

Critique and legacy of Taylorism

On the plus side, Taylor wanted to take the unnecessary toil out of work and believed that increased productivity would lead to a living wage. But he studied the bottom end of the hierarchy without being 'bottom-up' in his attitudes towards management control, putting the onus on the workers to make an organisation profitable without according them any status beyond the mechanistic. His methods gave no scope to imagination or innovation. Workers were treated as less than human and not as able to innovate or change their own working patterns for the better. Nevertheless, Taylor is remembered as the first person to study work as a subject in its own right.

Henry Ford

Some of the early, top-down managers certainly got things done. Ford (1863–1947), for example, was a genius at marketing. He paid his workers twice the going rate in order to turn them into a market for his own cars, and introduced mass production methods to keep up with the sales of an affordable, reliable and practical product that everybody wanted. Other modern touches we can recognise included special offers (a $20 refund promised, and delivered, to every purchaser in the country if sales hit a certain target) and international marketing efforts. By 1920, the Ford Motor Company was producing a car a minute and was the largest and most profitable manufacturing enterprise in the world. Ford never trusted managers, hung onto control himself and sacked anyone else who tried to make decisions; he saw no reason why one department in his business empire should know what another was doing and eventually lost a great deal of money. There are no real parallels in social work, although a few directors of social services have been good at marketing either their organisations or themselves.

Of more relevance to us is the recognition that, now we are post-modern, we are also post-Fordist. The assembly line in industry has been replaced by fragmented work groups, in fragmented locations, with fragmented careers. The advent of the telecottage, where the analyst or accountant works from home, is the epitome of this development. Although the trend is less evident in social work than in many other sectors, there are growing numbers of freelance trainers, consultants, mentors and other self-employed people using their social work qualifications and experience to work from home. Interestingly, post-Fordist, home-based working and 'hot desking' are also beginning to affect the organisation of social services, with a number of authorities deciding they can save money on unneces-sary office space if social workers work from home as much as possible, using laptops and teleworking, and access workstations in the nearest office rather than each having a separate desk in a fixed location and travelling miles back to base from each visit. All employers are seeking to improve record-keeping and budgetary control through computerisation, with electronic case files allowing managers to access information at any time and look for trends across cases. There are implications for user confidentiality as well as for the health and safety of workers (eye and muscle strain from using computers without workstation assessments, risk of violent theft of the laptop, stress induced by reduced clerical support and by the lack of colleague contact and teamwork). Post-Fordism is now a reality in social work and is bringing new challenges with it. Certainly, procedural efficiency, based on performance indicators and monitored outcomes, appears to have taken the place of build-ing relationships.

Summary of classical theories of management

To sum up, the study of management is rooted in the classical tendency to see organisations as machines and their employees as cogs, each carrying out one specialised task. Associated particularly with continuous processing and mass production, this model regards managers as holding top-down responsibility for planning, monitoring and motivating the work of others within their span of control. These ideas are now regarded by theorists as too rigid and predictable to reflect the contemporary world of work, yet there are certain echoes of them in the government's managerialist agendas for social services of standardised performance targets, league tables based on numerical measurements, and efficiency gains.

Organisational structures

Max Weber: the efficiency of bureaucracy

The name of Max Weber (1864–1920), a German sociologist, has become synonymous with the concept of bureaucracy, although he did not invent it. Rather, he formulated a typology of organisational forms, based on the exercise of power and authority (that is, the behaviour *within* organisations and not just their outward shape), from which the bureaucracy emerged as the most technically efficient. This does not mean that Weber found it attractive; indeed, he found it a rather terrifying vision of the future.

Weber's interest was in what makes people follow instructions. A leader, he concluded, may exercise *charismatic* authority through a combination of personal qualities and vision (unfortunately true of some abusive residential regimes, as well as religious and political movements), or may hold *traditional* authority on account of hereditary position. *Rational-legal authority*, Weber's third type, is that exercised within bureaucratic organisations and is the one that dominates in social work because the chief form of delivery is through large, local authority bureaucracies or voluntary organisations in which a high value is placed on personal and organisational accountability. In this model, the arbitrary power and influence of the founder of a business or political dynasty is missing. Rather, the conformity comes from following formalised rules and procedures, and working within clear-cut structures (which managers and practitioners may struggle to balance against the creativity and flexibility needed to respond to complex problems in people's lives).

Notably, Weber defined the bureaucratic organisational structure as a hierarchy of *offices,* or posts, rather than individuals. Each office carries specific responsibilities for which the person occupying it should have the relevant skills. This we would recognise as a job description (see Chapter 5). It means that the fundamental structure of a bureaucracy may be illustrated as a set of roles; each individual occupies a box within the structure, located in relation to the rest of the hierarchy. The design of this structure would look

Figure 2.1 Hierarchical structure

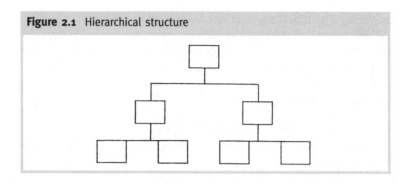

like that shown in Figure 2.1, which is basically a pyramid, with the head of the organisation at the top, middle managers in between and frontline workers and their assistants at the base. Typically, the bigger an organisation gets, the taller this pyramid becomes. This is one reason why 'downsizing' usually involves cutting out whole layers of deputy or middle managers.

Shorn of its emotional connotations (of over-rigid, mechanistic rule by paperwork), we can see that there are elements of bureaucracy in all formal organisations. According to Weber (1947), the five main characteristics of a 'pure' bureaucracy are:

1. A *clear-cut division of labour,* with activities rationally distributed as official duties (you work within your job description and on work as allocated, not what you feel like doing that day).
2. The distribution of duties through a *formal administrative hierarchy,* in which each office is supervised by the one above it and communication is required to pass up and down this supervisory chain. (A social worker does not just ring up the director to ask for more resources or advice on a difficult case, nor do people conduct their work through those they happen to get on with.)
3. A prescribed system of *rules and procedures,* which, if not followed, can lead to disciplinary action and, conversely, should safeguard the worker if the rules *are* followed but a case does not turn out well.
4. The exclusion of *personal considerations* from the conduct of official business, both by the employee and the organisation.

(Here, thinking has moved on somewhat, as we shall see below, but it is still absolutely the case that social workers must be able to distinguish between their personal and professional boundaries.)

5. Salaried employment based on *technical qualifications* and constituting a career within the hierarchy – recruitment and selection against job descriptions and person specifications, staff development and promotion prospects all relate to this element of a bureaucratic organisation.

Critique of the bureaucratic model in social work

This formalised, hierarchical model is still commonly found in social welfare organisations (albeit with elaborations – see below) and it does offer some benefits. There are undoubtedly advantages to a large workforce in having clear lines of command, coherence and predictable rules. The organisation is more readily answerable to those who use its services – in allocating resources fairly, for example – and also to staff members who may feel aggrieved. Workers know when they apply for promotion what abilities they will be expected to have and can usually expect staff development opportunities to assist them if they want to move on in their career because this is also to the advantage of the organisation. Some security is offered inasmuch as staff know who does what and that there is stability in the system.

There are also limitations for social work in this organisational form because:

1. It is best suited to *routine, stable, unchanging tasks.* Consequently, there have always been doubts about its appropriateness for social work practice. Not only is social work forever in a state of flux at the wider level, as thinking about social welfare changes along with the political climate but, at the front line, it also has to deal with the messiness and unpredictability of people's lives. This makes it hard to give anything but the most general indication of how each person should be treated, or, at the other extreme, risks turning people into categories and losing the social work skill of working with each as a unique individual in a specific set of circumstances. This is what some social workers fear is happening, for example, as they complete Assessment and

Action Records on looked after young people – as if a checklist of apparently objective judgements could adequately encompass the professional and ethical dilemmas involved in working with human diversity and agency (Garrett, 1999).

2. A rigid organisational structure is not well suited to situations where individual members of staff are required to exercise personal judgement or *professional autonomy* (Aldridge, 1996). Social workers are not expected to have to be told in detail how to do their jobs. They bring with them the ability to make specialised, individualised and complex judgements about people and their lives which is the hallmark of the qualified professional. Consequently, a hybrid term of 'bureau-professionalism' is sometimes used to apply to the social work context.

3. A rigid approach may be less responsive to the many, potentially *competing stakeholders* in social work beyond the immediate employing organisation. First, social workers retain more autonomy than factory-floor workers because they draw their professional skills, knowledge and values from outside points of reference (Mintzberg, 1989), particularly those of a university-based academic discipline and a professional association with its own ethical code (in the UK this is the British Association of Social Workers – BASW), as well as the requirements of a regulatory body (in England, the General Social Care Council, and, elsewhere, the Scottish Social Services Council, the Care Council for Wales and the Northern Ireland Social Care Council). These organisations are linked into global groupings of practitioners, teachers and researchers who are in continual debate about what social work is, what it can achieve and the standards by which it should operate. Second, those bodies that actually pay social workers' wages are themselves loosely grouped into an 'employers' lobby' consisting of many disparate organisations. There are also many other relevant groupings that are bigger and more influential than a single agency, from representative bodies such as the Association of Directors of Social Service to the 'benchmarking club' involving 20 councils in London through which managers decided to pool information on performance and establish baseline charges and standards (*Community Care*, 14–20 January 1999, p. 6). Third, there is increasing

pressure on social work, and rightly so, to be responsive to users and carers, as well as to the general public who feed their views, for example, into local community care plans.

4. The more diverse an organisation's activities and the more types of people it serves, the greater the *complexity* required in the shape that holds everything together (Haynes, 2003). Thus social services, for example, tends to sprout side shoots in the form of specialist teams or, increasingly, workers are outposted into multidisciplinary teams where staff from other agencies or professions, such as hospital consultants, managers of youth offending teams or teachers, will be as influential as the social workers' own departmental managers. Such structures are likely to become more common with the increase in partnerships with and within bodies such as Primary Care Trusts, Community Mental Health Trusts and Children's Trusts. Also, there is an increasing need for non-social work, technical specialists to manage or advise on whole parts of the organisation or department's activities, such as computing, legal or equalities issues. Their policy priorities and links with staff may cut across operational line management, that is, across the overseeing of the basic business of that department or agency. Similar complications exist in large voluntary organisations where the management of fundraising and policy development is as important as running the direct services provided. It is increasingly difficult for the manager in a complex public sector organisation to encompass this degree of diversity either in organisational structure or technical expertise. There have been, for example, some enormously expensive mistakes made in computer purchasing (notably in health settings), when managers have not known that they were being given bad advice.

Despite these complications, on paper at least, the up-and-down chain of accountability and delegation remains clear however many strata there are, although the level of responsibility and the boundaries around the roles at each level clearly differ. Nevertheless, there are, however, both formal and informal variations on the bureaucratic organisational form in and around social work:

1. Informally, as we shall see in a later section, *organisations are living entities* (Geus, 1997), in the sense that they are imbued

with the characteristics and interrelationships of the staff who people them. Weber's mechanistic charting of organisational structure does not display the way people 'bend the rules', circumvent their line managers or find themselves acting outside their role (for example domestic staff in group homes who are sought out for a personal 'chat' by the children living there and find themselves being asked for advice). People also 'act up' in their posts, either with or without official sanction, from the care organiser who is trusted beyond her actual responsibilities to the temporary senior covering leave or secondment. Interestingly, acting up has been found to be an important way in which women gain the confidence, experience and credibility to apply for management jobs (Allan et al., 1992; see Chapter 7). But it can also be a way in which some individuals and not others are groomed for promotion, and a means of exploiting the goodwill or insecurity of someone whose career development is not advanced accordingly.

2. There are some jobs, such as staff development officer, that always present difficulties in deciding where to *locate the post holders*. Are they in the senior management team or are they middle managers? Is their work part of strategic planning or can only the operational managers know how the changing nature of the work on the ground throws up new training needs? Ideally, they should be bringing together operational and strategic considerations, but this tends to put a strain on over-simple ideas about structure.

3. Overall, the hierarchical chart conveys no sense of *where an organisation is going* or what it is becoming over time, that is, of its 'organic' elements. With such a rapid pace of change in social work, restructuring has become the norm and organisational thinking has to be dynamic, not static.

4. There are a few clear exceptions to the hierarchical model of the pure bureaucracy that social workers may come across. It is important to recognise and value their difference:

   ● *Collectives* – Some organisations, usually small in size, operate as a collective, with shared decision-making, or a cooperative, which also implies shared ownership. In a women's refuge, for example, there may be a collective of workers, although less often than formerly (see Chapter 7).

They share tasks, are accountable to a wider grouping of women, often including service user representatives, rather than through a hierarchy and make the rules jointly with them. They value what workers who may themselves be survivors of men's violence can bring in personal as well as professional terms to their work, and they do not work their way up through a career structure. Where there are women designated as managers, this often tends to have been imposed as a condition of outside funding by people who assume that good management means managers.

● *Parallel hierarchies* – Other organisational variants that social work students may wish to consider can be found in hospitals and universities, where senior doctors and senior academics work in parallel hierarchies alongside senior administrators who are not equipped to question their medical or subject-based specialist knowledge in conducting an open-heart operation or marking an exam in Ancient Greek. Many pre-1992 universities also have elected heads of department, on a rotating basis, who may be junior (in promotion terms) to some of those for whom they hold many line management responsibilities. Increasingly, in both hospital and university settings, central management is becoming more powerful and there are also external moves to find ways of imposing verifiable standards, such as updating for doctors on evidence-based medicine or measures of 'graduateness' among students.

Human relations theorists

To Weber and Fayol, people were roles in a hierarchy of responsibilities; to Taylor, they were cogs in a machine; to Ford, the consumers of his products and the workers on his assembly lines. A reaction against these mechanistic approaches came in the form of the human relations movement. The key thinkers behind this approach recognised that people not only work for an organisation, they *are* the organisation. Of equal importance as the manifest formal structure is the informal structure created by the behaviour of people, as individuals and in groups, as they live out the unpredictabilities and emotional vagaries that social workers know so well.

Mary Parker Follett: human problems and working them out together

Mary Parker Follett (1868–1933) was instrumental in shifting the emphasis in management from a concern with organisational control to one of sensitivity to human factors. Active in social work in turn-of-the-century Boston, it was through establishing evening classes and youth employment bureaux that Follett came to study industry and management as a political scientist. She saw management as a dynamic concept where power must go with responsibility. Authority should be vested in knowledge and experience, wherever these were located in the organisation, not in mere position on a hierarchy. It required *consent*. Just like most social workers, she considered that management should be based on the ethical principle of respect for human worth and dignity, not the emotionally sterile pursuit of efficiency at any cost.

Through her interest in people, Follett recognised that workers and managers often do not have a common aim and that, within teams and other work groups, there may be a good deal of conflict. In what we would now recognise as turning every threat into an opportunity (see Chapter 4), Follett believed that a group working together could air each person's viewpoint and build the best from each into an idea that no one would have been able to see on their own (Follett, 1925). Not only might this lead to a better overall solution, but it would not depend on one side winning over the other or an untidy compromise.

Follett drew her thinking about the worth of all people and the dynamic integration of organisations into four fundamental principles which are still relevant today:

1. To achieve coordination, it is important that people, regardless of their position, should have *direct contact with one another*. Horizontal communication is as important as vertical.
2. Everyone concerned with a policy or decision should be involved *from the early stages*. They should not be brought in afterwards as this denies the benefits of participation, increased motivation and raised morale.
3. Coordination depends on seeing all factors in a situation as *inter-related*.
4. Coordination and executive decisions are *continuing processes*; nothing is final. And, because so many people contribute to a

decision, it is an illusion to suggest that, ultimately, the person in the hierarchy who carries the authority is the one and only person on whom responsibility can be placed.

Although Follett believed in the essentials of leadership – the ability to see and understand the organisation and its context in their entirety and to have a vision of the future – she did not accept either the cult of the leader or the right of leaders to assume they know best or to set themselves above the rest. For her, the managerial vision should flow from the common purpose and the shared work and aspirations of the whole group. She sought to integrate the core tensions of management, such as the balance between the need to be rational and systematic while also being empathic and flexible, themes now seen as visionary in their time and taken up in more recent management literature (see, for example, Zander and Zander, 2000).

Elton Mayo: motivating people

Just as people can affect the working of a system, so too can they be affected by it, that is, by the general climate in the workplace and the way they are treated there. Elton Mayo's (1880–1949) research revealed that every organisation has an informal structure which affects how people behave, how the system functions and which management methods need to be adopted to raise morale and assist people to be mentally healthy at work. His importance lay in drawing attention to all the other aspects of motivation and productivity beyond the purely financial, which was all that Taylor believed made people work to their full capacity.

Mayo saw that business methods that take no account of wider human issues, such as emotional reactions and the social climate of the workplace, can lead first to subtle sabotage and then to formalised industrial conflict. He was ahead of his time, too, in seeing the need to adapt to rapid changes both in technology and society. He believed in explaining change to the workforce and taking their attitudes into account when introducing it (see the section in Chapter 3 on the management of change).

Mayo is best known for the research he undertook for the Western Electric Company of Chicago – the 'Hawthorne' studies. The company's aim was to undertake objective, scientific studies of performance in a factory setting to evaluate which variables improved output. They intended to evaluate the differences in performance between a target group given new ways of working and a control group that continued as before. The unexpected finding of the Hawthorne experiments was that *both* groups improved their productivity during the research. This inspired one of the best-known terms in the study of motivation and performance, the 'Hawthorne effect', meaning the tendency of people to change their behaviour simply because they are being paid attention, in this case being subjected to social investigation, regardless of the context or intention. It also highlighted the crucial understanding that people respond better when other people, managers, researchers or whoever, take a serious and genuine interest in what they are doing, something organisations of all kinds can still fail to remember.

Through observing the behaviour of small working groups in the same company over more than a decade from 1924, Mayo explored the informal social systems which grow up among employees and which, because they underlie both cooperation and resistance to change, must play a part in the effective organisation of work. People have a natural propensity to associate with one another and they care what 'their' group thinks about them. To be motivated, they need a management style that maintains and builds on this spontaneous cooperation in groups, takes a genuine interest in both the individual and the group, provides new interest from time to time and also recognises that workers, employed in an enterprise which has been artificially created to achieve certain ends, do think about what good their work is to the wider society. All this makes perfect sense in social work.

Chris Argyris

Argyris (1923–) suggested that workers do not grow or become self-actualised in structures which offer them little control over their work. Rather, people who do not experience autonomy and involvement adapt their behaviour in ways that are immature, passive and dependent (1957). Initiative is lacking, people 'clock watch', take longer and longer breaks, cling to habitual routines, resist change, impede progress and show minimal commitment to the agency or its work. Management responds with repressive control, staff grow yet more infantilised and resistant and a downward spiral is created that, unfortunately, is not unknown in social work settings. If it were possible to encourage ways of working that did not put individual and organisational needs in opposition, then Argyris considered that worker satisfaction and productivity might both improve.

His model of management takes a multidimensional view of a worker as not just a strong arm or a good mind but a *whole person*. Organisations are made up of people and managers need to think about the way they conceptualise, and hence treat, the people they employ – the extent to which workers' personal and social needs are met. This model is, then, a more 'organic' one than those in the classical tradition. It emphasises the unplanned aspects of the organisation, such as employee morale and motivation (seen as naturally present and therefore only needing channelling), informal social groups, an individual's need for job enrichment as well as good pay and the way teams might control, collaborate and participate in task achievement. Information gathered through routine monitoring and evaluation would be used, not to check up on people, but to help people in their activities. Managers at the top would increase their interpersonal competence by being honest and showing their real feelings according to this view.

Douglas McGregor

McGregor (1906–1964) another psychologist, built on Abraham Maslow's (1954) motivation theory of basic human needs, with which many social workers will be familiar. Once basic physiological and safety needs have been met, people at work become interested in *self-fulfilment and responsibility*. So work is not just a source of money but of self-respect, risk-taking and creativity (contrast the way that Taylor thought about his workers). If this is so, then positions have to be designed and fitted to people in the hierarchy, rather than the other way round.

McGregor (1960) coined the terms 'Theory X' and 'Theory Y' to describe the authoritarian and participative approaches to management. An organisation based on Theory X would assume that people are naturally lazy, irresponsible and resistant, rather than being made that way by the organisation they work in. Managers would have to assign tasks and, like Taylor, be job-centred rather than person-centred; supervisors would ensure that their subordinates were kept busy. The design of the organisation would be one of clear lines of authority, narrow spans of control and centralised decision-making.

On the other hand, the organisational implications of Theory Y, where people are naturally striving, taking pride in their accomplishments and seeking new experiences, would indicate a structure which delegates responsibility and control, encouraging workers to *participate* in decision-making. Some social services agencies still manage to operate in this style and consider that it is easier to meet quality standards when staff are committed to their work and the organisation is not dogged by uncontrolled sick leave, high staff turnover or low morale (see Chapter 6). Joint Reviews of local authority social services have found that the organisations that serve local people best are also the ones that involve and invest in their staff (Jones, 2000). Theory Y-style management certainly seems more suited to social work and social care.

Rensis Likert

Likert (1903–1981) was always interested in leadership styles. He actually asked employees in US companies how they were treated (it was from his attitude research that he gave his name to the 'Likert scale', which grades responses to survey questions) and, in a 1961 book based on this research, categorised four systems of organisational management along a continuum from exploitative and authoritarian, through benevolent authoritative, to consultative and finally participative (Likert, 1961). Although he found the benevolent authoritative management system to be the most common at the time, he favoured the *participative* style as most successful in the longer term. A close-knit work group (see Figure 2.2) which

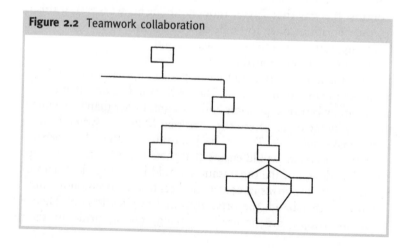

Figure 2.2 Teamwork collaboration

supports management's aims can, he thought, induce its members to be more efficient, just as a resistant one can pull performance down.

On the other hand, a team which forgets that it is still part of its employing organisation, and which uses its collaborative strength to deviate from organisational norms or purposes, is likely to find itself pulled back into line. To avoid this, the leaders of effective work groups not only get to know people as individuals and allow maximum participation in decision-making, but also ensure that the group's contributions are linked to the overall performance of the organisation. These managers need to function as 'linking pins' between the group they manage and the management group. In other words, they need to think of themselves as members of both groups because they constitute the primary communications chain within the organisation. When drawn on an organisation chart, the manager is a linking pin at the top of a triangle, the base of which is formed by his/her team (see Figure 2.3).

The downside of this is, of course, that middle managers may feel like the meat in the sandwich – hemmed in from both sides as they try to respond to ever increasing team and management pressure (each of which may in turn be operating under wider ranging influence such as government regulation, user and carer demands or trade union views). The team leader will know exactly how that feels!

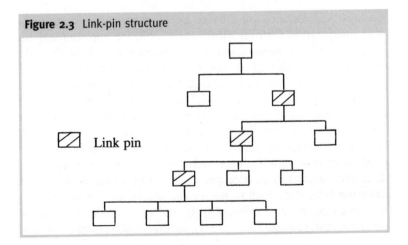

Figure 2.3 Link-pin structure

Link pin

Critique of the human relations school

The great strength of the human relations theorists is to have demonstrated the major impact that social factors have on work behaviour. This impact is so strong, whether for good or ill, that organisations need to build on the motivation of the personnel they employ both by valuing each individual and building cooperation in teams. The efforts of the later human relations theorists, such as Argyris, McGregor and Likert, naturally became increasingly sophisticated and demonstrated that the relationships between intrinsic job satisfaction, group morale and output were more complicated than simply being happy at work and being part of a cooperative work group. There were key elements of management style and structure, as these related to the workforce, that could have a profound effect. Even so, critics felt that some of the research led to unrealistic conclusions, such as the idea of handing over all problem-solving to work groups lower down the organisation.

An overall criticism of this body of work is that, although these theorists have drawn on psychology, sociology, philosophy and anthropology, they remain located within business studies and centrally concerned with the productivity needs of organisations. At the end of the day, this is still about controlling work, not about personal issues or interpersonal relations for their own sake; it is almost as if aspects of people's humanity are being understood only to be used against them so as to turn them into more compliant workers. And, since people are seen as being there to serve the needs of industry rather than the other way round, the approach cannot be good at asking the big questions. Does our society have the right organisations, undertaking the right work, or might some of people's resistance within their employment settings be the result of dissatisfaction at this wider level? This can certainly be the case in social welfare where social workers and others are involved in major debates about the overall nature and aims of the welfare state, well beyond the details of practice. Thus, while the recognition of the need for good human relations might be a more congenial approach than the authoritarian concepts of scientific managerialism, the intention behind it is still to pursue the aim of any organisation to be more effective and efficient in its use of resources and, in the private sector, to ensure a return on the investment. In other words, to make worker satisfaction and increased productivity complement each other through collaboration.

Nevertheless, it is all to the good that, as rationality and bureaucracy have proved inadequate concepts to meet the appropriate efficiency imperative in organisations, greater interest has begun to be shown in 'softer' concepts such as culture, emotions and gender (Hearn and Parkin, 1995). The human messiness that the Weberian legacy viewed as 'inimical to rational, efficient capitalism' has now become an essential part of theorising about organisations (Clegg, 1990, p. 150). Social workers are on home ground with such thinking, of course, for example in Thompson's (2003) writing about informal worker resistance to oppressive organisational cultures.

The organisation becoming more complex: the systems model

As we saw in the last section, more sophisticated thinkers have increasingly come to see that organisations are made up of people and that this greatly affects what happens in them. Systems thinking had a similar genesis. In the period before and after the Second World War, a number of academic disciplines became interested in how inanimate as well as animate organisms work as systems moving from consideration of the brain to newly developing computers and thence to business organisations and other large institutions. The key ideas were that each organisation is both a system itself and made up of other systems, all systems tend towards an internal equilibrium, and organisations are 'open' systems in that they interact with their environment.

Eric Trist: origins of the organisational model

At the Tavistock Institute of Human Relations in London, Eric Trist (1911–1993) and his colleagues developed a theory of 'open systems' which recognises the dynamic movement in and out of organisations as well as inside them. Classical models had been constructed from observing virtually closed business systems, usually pursuing specific economic goals, and had left out the 'people factors' as well as the external context. Organisations, though, employ and serve human beings and also operate in turbulent, ever changing fields where the outside world can be as influential as policy made internally (in social work, think of media scandals over child deaths, or government changes in welfare legislation).

When Trist and his colleagues studied the effects of mechanisation on the Durham coal mines, what is interesting to social workers is that they realised they had to put the people into the equation. They found that, if an organisation was to operate effectively, *its technical systems had to mesh with its social systems*. Technology had disturbed miners' small and semi-autonomous shift groupings. As a result, social stress occurred, with resultant absenteeism, scapegoating and defensiveness. (It is interesting that both high rates of sick leave and the negative impact of a 'culture of blame' were in the news in social work at the height of the influence of 'managerialism', leading managers to rediscover that they needed to work with employees as people.)

Trist showed that the organisation of work has social and psychological properties of its own, that is, that social and technical systems interact. In particular, he demonstrated the role of motivation in productivity and team-building. Unlike robots, people find satisfaction in finishing a whole task, controlling their own behaviour, setting their own targets and in working together as a team; a comprehensive assessment, for example, is a complex piece of work in which a sophisticated professional judgement is balanced against that of other professionals, the views of users and carers, and the policies and resource allocations of the employing organisation. These insights are being rediscovered as practitioners increasingly find that merely inputting information into computers, without the opportunity to use their wider social work skills, is not only dissatisfying but also ineffective. The recognition that work can be an immensely satisfying part of life, when well organised and fulfilling, also reminds us that unemployment and 'underemployment' among excluded groups, such as disabled people (Oliver and Barnes, 1998) and asylum seekers, is still a challenge that our society is failing to meet.

Key concepts in thinking about organisations as systems

The systems approach does not prescribe any particular organisational design. Rather, it is a way of understanding the structure an organisation already happens to have, the processes that go on within that structure, and the way that changing particular interactions might help it work better towards its desired outcomes.

Systems theory offers us a number of concepts which may be relevant in thinking about organisations. Each organisation can itself be conceptualised as a system, by analogy with a biological system such as the human body. This means that:

- it has *boundaries* around it
- it is composed of *subsystems* – in the body's case, these include the circulatory and respiratory systems, and in social services they include information and financial systems
- it interacts with other discrete systems in *super-systems* – people interact with each other in societies; organisations interact with each other, for example, in a wider system of welfare, encompassing health, social care, housing, financial support and so on.

Confusingly, we tend to use the word 'system' in professional speech for a subsystem ('finance system') or for a super-system ('system of welfare') more readily than for the discrete system itself, the organisation. This is probably because in the first two cases we have to make an effort to conceptualise all the financial arrangements or all the welfare agencies working together, whereas we always think of the organisation as one defined entity. In this section, we will describe all three types just as 'systems' but we need to remember that they overlap and coexist in a range of ways.

The boundaries around a system may be more or less open or permeable or they may be closed. A body's respiratory system is open to the air being sucked in and pushed out; the circulatory system of the blood is permeable to the oxygen extracted while the air is in the body. These two subsystems working together help the body to maintain its energy levels and thereby its total functioning. In an organisation, we may speak of an information system being open to those who record material in it or look up that material; it may become open to a new set of people, such as service users, if they are given rights to see their files, or if details about the agency's decisions begin to be published. The information itself is part of what the organisation needs to carry out its work, like oxygen in the body.

What happens inside systems

The analogy between breathing and using information can also be used to understand the terms applied to energy use by systems:

- *input* – the energy being *fed into the system across the boundary* (breathing in air; gathering information)

- *throughput* – the use made of the energy *inside the system* (oxygen extracted in the lungs, passed into the blood and circulated round the body to help create warmth and movement; information recorded and used to decide what type of assessment or individual care plan is needed)
- *output* – the energy passing *back out of the system into the environment* (breathing out carbon dioxide; publishing statistics on the services devoted to individual care plans over a 12-month period).

There is a further process whereby output loops back on itself to affect input and throughput:

- *feedback loop* – a health check-up might test exhalation to judge the state of the lungs; a care agency, looking back over reviews of care plans and people's responses to them, may in turn alter what care managers do in constructing future plans.

'Healthy open systems must devote part of their resources to monitoring the impact of their outputs on their environment' (Chetkow-Yanoov, 1992, p. 25) and, certainly, social work organisations would aim to use monitoring information to improve their work. Current thinking about performance is aimed at ensuring that this information includes service users' views about the services they receive. A simple diagram of this input, throughput and output – happening in the operation of a welfare agency – is shown in Figure 2.4.

As mentioned above, it is important not to forget the people

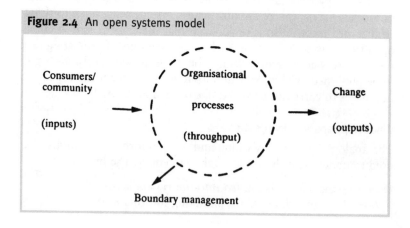

Figure 2.4 An open systems model

Consumers/
community

(inputs)

Organisational

processes

(throughput)

Change

(outputs)

Boundary management

within the system. For Senge (1992), for example, systems thinking is what links together the human potential within an organisation to build a shared vision, model fresh alternatives, learn new ways of working as a team and see how their own actions impede or create change. The staff in a health or social care organisation, just as in a large corporation, can generate a wholly new approach to service delivery if their combined efforts can facilitate a fundamental shift in the established ways of thinking and doing things. A particular benefit of thinking in whole systems is that it allows managers to cope with change by raising their preoccupations beyond the detail of day-to-day work to engage with other organisations and the rest of the external environment (Haynes, 2003).

Systems thinking in social work and care management

Systems theory has always had a special place in social work because it encompasses both ideas on practice, notably in family therapy, and ways of managing the whole organisation (Bilson and Ross, 1999). The manager's key role in the systems approach is to focus on how the subsystem(s) he or she manages relate(s) at all the points of 'interface' with the larger, total system and the outside world – known as 'boundary management'. (This is very different from earlier thinking, which saw managers as being there to solve internal conflicts.) The systems approach relates well to care management, for example, because the latter emphasises the crucial links between commissioners and a range of external and in-house providers, as well as the important interlinking between all the different parts of the organisation that deal with quality standards, complaints, contracting, budgets and so on, and other external bodies such as housing and health authorities.

Perhaps the missing element for care managers, as the role has developed in many authorities, is the freedom really to be managers of these interfaces – to construct imaginative care packages drawing on a wide range of informal carers and formal care providers (including writing their own skills into contracts), rather than the somewhat uniform responses that often apply, and to handle all the complex communications involved. If all social workers are managers, as suggested in Chapter 1, then these tasks are certainly encompassed by social work skills, and groups of care managers working together in teams could get more involved in juggling budgets and thinking about the standards needed in contracts for services.

Critique of the systems model

Although systems approaches are an improvement on the over-simplistic classical models, they are still only artificial attempts to capture the complexities of the real world and, despite the use of 'organic' language, the approach is somewhat pseudoscientific, with no allowance for human emotions. Systems analysis provides an abstract description but can never lay down a strategy or guide for action or behaviour. Other theories are needed for that. The model is also artificially politically neutral, functionalist and normative, taking little or no account of the *interplay of power dynamics* within the organisation, including where there may be racist, sexist or other oppressive elements built into the systems or the aims of the organisation, as well as inherent in the attitudes of particular staff.

Like any theoretical model, systems theory is only an attempt to look at something essentially familiar in fresh ways. It does not exist in reality, so it can mislead us, and it can get in the way of other ideas. For example, the analogy with biological bodies is not at all exact. Two organisations could decide to share a subsystem (a post-adoption or out-of-hours service, for example, or health and social services undertaking joint commissioning) without losing their distinctive identity. If we worked too closely to the agency/human body parallel, we could overlook some important possibilities for working in partnership.

Most worryingly, systems analysis may be a force for unhealthy conservatism. It does not cope well with the 'big questions'. For example, a system such as a corrupt or bankrupt organisation may actually need to lose some of its parts or dissolve altogether. The model contains no clear place for political questions such as how the system came to be the way it is, who holds the most power within or over it, why some systems suck in more energy (resources, personal information) than they can put to good use, who decides what constitutes 'good use' – or how fundamental inequities, such as poverty and racism, can ever be radically opposed by systems which have been created in their image and typically operate to sustain them. In using a systems analysis to look at organisations, we need to take care not to ignore these bigger questions of power and powerlessness.

To sum up, as organisations have become bigger and more

complex, the systems model has attempted to offer a manageable way of thinking about them, as if they were giant bodies, with all their activities interacting. Everything connects to everything else and it is in the interactions, and at the boundaries where they take place (internally and externally), that change can happen. Social workers are traditionally attracted by the ideas of openness, teamwork and interdependence in systems thinking. They also like the fact that a theory they may have learned for social work practice or systemic family therapy can double up for use in understanding organisations (Coulshed and Orme, 1998).

The model has served us well in encouraging managers to think about what inputs will produce the desired outputs and, with a dynamic sense, about processes of development and change. It is being outdone now, however, by the sheer complexity of the scope and inner workings of many organisations. The loosely coupled system refers to the various subsystems as now virtually independent, each needing to be understood on its own terms in order to understand the whole (Leigh, 1988). When SSDs were still unified entities, for example, children's provider services, children's commissioning, adult provider services and care management all came to operate increasingly separately until, in many parts of the UK, they split apart entirely. Some elements of the work have been 'outsourced' to contractors and private tenderers, thus adding a further layer of complication.

Where are we now? Complexity and the challenge of constant change

So fast has the rate of change become in organisations and so complex their structure, that none of the above historical models is now considered adequate to understand or manage them. A whole new set of models of organisational structure that attempts to grapple with this layer of complexity will be outlined in Chapter 4.

Because of the challenges of the task, especially in terms of the networks required to deliver change and the tendency to specialisation and fragmentation within organisations, the role of the organisation's leaders emerged as a focal point for organisational purpose, survival and identity. It came to be seen as critically important for the relevant director to hold everything together – enthusing all the staff with an overall vision and a shared culture and values, imbuing the organisation with a corporate image and managing the changes necessary to cope with new challenges and demands. Chapters 3 and 4 will look at these issues of culture and change, vision and mission, as key aspects of management thinking in the 1990s. Since then, models of management, like other social sciences in the UK, have come under the influence of complexity theory. The sheer unpredictability of constant change has led to a certain scepticism about rational decision-making and top-down leadership. The ensuing chapters will also deal, therefore, with the move beyond the rational towards the more imaginative and creative in management theory.

3 | Cultural change and quality standards

As we saw in Chapter 2, management and organisational theory moved from abstract model-building to understanding the workforce as human beings rather than as cogs in a machine. Paradoxically, organisations can become more efficient if, instead of trying to tidy the people in them into neat little pigeonholes and control their every action, human needs are responded to and human strengths – creativity, enthusiasm, engagement – are fostered. In social work, as elsewhere, this has to happen in a context of constant change which can create enormous uncertainty and even hostility. This means there is quite a challenge facing the managers who must provide the leadership to motivate staff under difficult circumstances and manage the process of change.

In the business world, meanwhile, another body of people has also come to the fore, that is, the customers who have to be attracted to consume goods and services through careful product design and marketing. In social work, too, quality services and value for money are seen as essential ways of meeting the needs of the consumer. Such matters can be looked at only within a broader approach to the whole culture of the organisation and its overall mission. Consequently, we will start with a consideration of these before moving on to quality and the management of change.

Culture

Organisations, like national and ethnic groupings, have a pervasive culture, and can also have subcultures within them that support or resist the dominant way of thinking. This culture – 'the way things are done here' – can be positive, as in a 'culture of excellence', or essentially negative, as in the tendency in social work towards a 'culture of blame'. Here, hostile media coverage, lack of political and public support, and scapegoating when something goes wrong lead employees to fear failure and care more about 'covering their backs' than about giving a good service (see also Chapter 6). At the same time, there are examples of social services organisations that have overcome negative and cynical cultures and now project pride and excitement in their work, a willingness to experiment and a commitment to mutual support.

McKenna and Beech (1995, p. 51, drawing on Hofstede, 1980) list some of the variations in national cultures that can also be seen in organisations. They express these in terms of low or high degrees of the following:

- *Power distance*: how autocratic the leaders are and the extent to which subordinates are trusted.
- *Uncertainty avoidance*: how willing people are to take risks, bend the rules, change jobs.
- *Individualism–collectivism*: Western individualism as against loyalty to family and community, the supportive workplace and the corporation.
- *Masculinity–femininity*: competitive ambition as against net-working, caring, bringing out the best in others (see Chapter 7).

Handy (1993), an influential management thinker, offered a different but overlapping listing of four types of organisational culture: *power culture* (strong leadership from a small group at the top), *role culture* (clinging to bureaucratic roles, rules and regulations), *task culture* (emphasising technical know-how, project teams) and *person culture* (matching tasks to people). Different cultures suit different types and sizes of organisation. They may also vary from one part of an organisation to another, although it is considered part of the management role to get the whole organisation pulling together.

The current trend is to try and change the organisational culture to one that is more likely to lead to success, with greater emphasis on trust and participation, managed risk, corporate loyalty, teamwork and good staff care. The aim is to make an organisation's structure and culture serve its overall strategy – what it is trying to achieve over time. However, giving attention to structure or culture alone can result in an inward-looking enterprise, where the needs and interests of service users get lost and in which nobody has a clear sense of purpose or direction. A clear vision and strategy from the top are also essential.

The interest in corporate culture arose initially from wondering why some nations' businesses were doing particularly well – first Japan in the 1980s and then the 'tiger economies' of Southeast Asia, until the near collapse of the financial markets adversely affected them all in the late 1990s. Among the factors thought to explain the earlier success were corporate loyalty and a commitment to quality shared by all, which we shall explore below, and investment in the selection and training of a stable workforce, which will feature in Chapters 5 and 6. Although only some aspects of the approach could be transplanted to the West, where social norms are different, there began to be seen greater interest in people, more emphasis on the group and teamworking, and more understanding that trust and participation can lead to better results, not loss of control.

An American response to the search for successful management practices able to create the right organisational culture was Peters and Waterman's *In Search of Excellence* (1982). They considered what was special about some of the USA's most successful companies, where the best was brought out in staff and an unparalleled service given to customers. Their book shifted attention to the importance of leadership and human resource management (HRM) and was influential across all sectors in the UK, although not without its critics (Salaman, 1992). The ideas were incorporated into central government's approach to public sector management, including in relation to social services. Peters and Waterman were timely and enthusiastic rather than rigorous in their approach, but some of their ideas have had a major impact, such as advocating:

- *action and decisiveness* from management, not endless reports and committees
- *staying close to the customer*, listening to them so as to understand and respond to their need for quality, service and reliability
- *autonomy and entrepreneurship*, with many smaller companies competing against each other more inclined to take risks in new directions than a few large and more cautious corporations tend to be
- *productivity through people*, where everyone's efforts count and everyone shares the rewards

- *hands-on managers,* in touch with the staff, who are driven by clearly defined values
- sticking to what the company *knows best and can do well*
- *simple, lean structures,* with fewer layers and fewer managers
- tight adherence to *fundamental organisational values,* controlled from the centre, with greater autonomy for staff in other regards, that is, through operational decentralisation.

During the 1990s, national and local political leaders and social work management tended to favour structural change as the main vehicle for service improvement, unfortunately the most contentious of the Peters and Waterman principles. Improvements in services were assumed to be more likely to occur in a competitive welfare market, in which SSDs shed many of their provider functions or organised them separately from commissioning (Walsh, 1995). The structural change to achieve this was often accompanied by managerial reorganisations in which layers of managers were reduced and a number of people were made redundant.

There was also a growing interest in the service user as 'customer', able to exercise power to achieve service improvement through choice. Care managers were expected to complete 'needs-led assessments' that identified the user's and carer's needs and wishes in each case and then put together packages of care, possibly from a number of providers, to meet those needs. This was in contrast to 'service-led assessments', which assessed people to see which council service they were most suited to, said to be what most social workers had done in the past. Nevertheless, budget realities still intrude on the needs-led approach so this may not equate, despite all, with meeting customer preferences.

Peters and Waterman began the shift away from managers seeing all the answers in abstract organisational structures, towards the 'new managerialist' or 'new wave management' focus on the people factors of staff and customers. At the same time, they did consider that organisational culture and success could be measured, in factors ranging from absenteeism to reputation (for customer care or equal opportunities, for example), and translated into performance indicators. This latter approach has arguably taken over in UK social work and social care, expressed by government in the language of quality but frequently emphasising top-down regulation over bottom-up autonomy and initiative. This may actually mean that key elements of the excellence findings are lost from sight. The impetus towards the development of occupational standards and professional competences, and government commitment to monitoring against performance indicators and national frameworks of standards, does not equate with the centre keeping hold of key values while decentralised operations are free to innovate and take risks.

The belief that excellence lies in the characteristics of managers and the culture they develop and sustain, as much as in those of the overall organisation, is reflected in a range of programmes and schemes introduced by the Local Government Association, the then Social Services Inspectorate and others to develop social services' managers. Evidence to support this has been found by external observers (Joint Reviews, 2004). There is also no doubt that government sees effective managers as key allies in the drive to improve services.

Quality

Overall approaches: quality control and quality assurance

The quest for high quality services can give rise to two contrasting images: either management checking up on the workforce or a collective effort to give the best possible service. These two approaches can be summed up as *quality control* and *quality assurance*.

Quality control, at its narrowest, implies looking at standards after the event and taking measures to rectify mistakes and stop them happening again. A somewhat broader version, which is becoming the norm in local government, involves *continually checking services against agreed standards*. It is a top-down model and certainly in tune with managerialist approaches. Every organisation needs an element of quality control (although it is not enough on its own, as we shall consider below). No single social work practitioner or manager can achieve significant improvements alone. Even if they attempt to raise the standards of their practice, they cannot judge whether they have succeeded unless they are part of wider-scale monitoring and feedback procedures with an agreed baseline of standards (Darvill, 1998b).

Quality assurance has more of an air of putting measures into effect in advance which will ensure that a *better and constantly improving job of work* is done. It is a more proactive approach, taken in the belief that 'You cannot inspect quality into a service' (Dunnachie, 1992, p. 19). Quality assurance is a bottom-up concept and tends to start from making the staff feel more involved so that they will pass this on in a better service to the consumers. This does tend to require a culture change in many organisations, not least in respect of involving care staff who have traditionally been accorded low pay and low status. If domestic and residential care workers are regarded as unskilled manual workers, doing 'women's work' that is not real work at all (see Chapter 6), they are less likely to be effectively drawn into the process of assuring quality.

Adams (1998) suggests a wider range of models: *quality rectification, quality maintenance, quality enhancement* and *quality maximisation*. (The first pair are effectively subdivisions of quality control and the second pair of quality assurance.) As the names suggest, quality rectification is error-driven; it implies responding only to complaints, adverse audits, investigations and inquiries, and whistleblowing (Hunt, 1998). Quality maintenance is standards-driven; it involves a more systematic approach to quality control but is based on achieving minimum standards, not on envisioning the ideal approach to service delivery, and it imposes standards largely set by 'experts', either in the form of the organisation's own managers or an external body.

Quality enhancement and quality maximisation are forms of quality assurance. Quality enhancement goes beyond minimum standards into setting goals that lead to continual improvement; it embraces quality management systems such as TQM (see below), which do involve a culture change (see Chapter 6) because people need to start listening to each other, but it does not question the overall approach to service delivery or the existing power relations within or beyond the organisation. Quality maximisation is, for Adams, an *empowerment model* that changes organisational culture more fundamentally, to embrace listening equally to all the stakeholders, including the collective voice of users. This could mean recognising, for example, that no standards, however high, will ever make professionally determined care packages as acceptable to many disabled people as services they can select and purchase for themselves, with the right to a social life perhaps featuring as importantly as personal care (Priestley, 1998).

An error-driven model may look the cheapest because it involves the least change but it is not. There are always costs involved in making mistakes and then rectifying them. These include the costs of dealing with complaints and, in extreme cases, being taken to court or to the local government ombudsman, perhaps paying compensation or having to hold an inquiry. Added to this are both the intangible costs of developing a poor reputation, so that future work becomes more difficult on many fronts, and the long-term costs of not providing preventive services so that problems intensify and replicate themselves over time. It is generally more cost-effective to get things right, even allowing for offering the improved service and monitoring its quality. Over and above all this, in social work and social care, we must never underestimate the human costs involved in failing to provide a good enough service at the time it is needed.

Quality standards

Before quality can be measured, there needs to be a general understanding of what it is. In everyday language, 'quality' goods and services often mean luxury ones, for which people who can afford to do so are prepared to pay more. In social work as in other public services, however, quality services are neither always the most expensive nor those that service users would necessarily choose; after all, many families would prefer not to have child care social workers involved at all and people in receipt of care packages might well want more than can equitably be provided. Rather, they are services that are fit for their purpose and reasonable in cost, with a degree of informed choice available wherever possible.

Thinking about cost has moved on. Under the Conservatives, the move towards compulsory competitive tendering (CCT) implied going for the cheapest option. Under New Labour, however, this was replaced by a move towards 'Best Value', meaning the achievement of the most advantageous combination of cost and quality (DETR, 1998, and see below). In determining 'quality', a duty is placed on local authorities to consult local people on service aims and standards, for example providing appropriate services for diverse communities. This includes those who use services and also local taxpayers, who ultimately pay for them. There are, in fact, a number of 'customers' and 'stakeholders' (other parties with an interest) who may need to be involved in setting quality standards.

In addition to users and their families, these include the general public, elected members on local authority committees and boards of trustees or management committees, and central government. Each has a different, if overlapping, set of interests that must be borne in mind by those responsible for writing quality standards.

A statement of standards must be approved by some of these groups and broadly acceptable to others. It must also be couched in specifics, outlining precisely what is to be achieved, to what level of performance, and how this will be measured. The last aspect is particularly important. A standard is insufficiently precise if we are not going to know when we have achieved it.

Anyone who has studied research methods will realise the complexity that this implies. In the social sciences, it is all too easy to slip into measuring only the *quantitative* elements of a service (for example how many meals are provided, of what nutritional value, at what cost) because this information is relatively easy to collate and compare. The national standards for mental health services in England and Wales and their performance indicators, for example, have gone for what is measurable and evidence-based, leaving the less tangible, more qualitative issues out of account and thereby discounting much of what social work does best (*Professional Social Work*, February 1999, p. 3). Most social work services, in fact, need to ask subjective and process-related questions, such as the extent to which users feel in control of their lives, able to influence the services they receive and treated as a person by staff (Qureshi, 1998). There is an additional complication in terms of all the people whose views may be relevant in assessing outcomes, just as they are in setting standards – not only users and carers, but also a range of agencies at different levels, those funding the service and so on.

Just because it is complicated does not mean, however, that no effort should be made to measure less tangible standards. This might be done in two stages. An initial questionnaire survey of all users, a series of meetings with residents or focus groups with representative users, for example, might reveal what factors people consider most important in the services they receive. These might then be usable as specific measures of quality. For example, consumers of meals on wheels might want not only a hot, nutritious meal, delivered on time and with a varied menu (all easy to measure), but also the opportunity to exchange a few words with the person delivering the meal.

This could be built into the timing of delivery rotas and measured by sampling user feedback. It is important not to confine users to a limited set of options as to what constitutes quality at this first stage because those options would come from our thinking, not theirs. A user group of adults with learning difficulties, for example, gave feedback that they did not consider professionals being smartly dressed to be a standard that was important to them; indeed, they associated people in suits with those who had deprived them of liberty and choices in earlier life. To them, the way people treated one another was far more important than how they looked.

Measuring outcomes

Once it has been decided what to measure, there are as many ways of doing so as there are of conducting research. In addition to the gathering and use of all possible forms of quantitative data, methods of measuring qualitative outcomes include an audit of records, a questionnaire survey, in-depth interviews with a sample of users, focus groups, or non-participant observation of the service while it is being delivered (Ellis and Whittington, 1998). There can also be routine user feedback built into the way the work is actually conducted, for example user comments in reviewing care plans and in residents' reviews, or simple surveys administered by those delivering the services. Levels of unmet demand in the community might be ascertained through community access points, freephone telephone lines, reply-paid cards, councillors' surgeries or commissioned public opinion research. Levels of response, of frankness in replies and of breadth of coverage will vary according to the method used.

Possible outcomes to measure include: user satisfaction; user knowledge of services; achievement of intended changes in users' attitudes, behaviour or quality of life; and users' ability to cope without further services. Clearly, the desirable outcome is dependent on the setting and user group. In some contexts (for example mental health), it might be a sign of failure, for example, if some people did not feel able to return for further help when they needed it, whereas in others, such as adopting children or leaving care, it tends to be hoped that people will be launched onto a path of living life unaided.

Although far from easy to arrive at, outcome standards are too general by themselves and need further work to express them in the form of indicator statements. Ellis and Whittington (1998) emphasise that these must be SMART: Specific, Measurable, Achievable,

Relevant and Targeted (others use the 'T' to refer to the need to work within set time limits, preferring the last term in the list to be Timed or Time-bound). An example they give of a generally desirable outcome is that of enabling the tenants of a supported housing scheme to make decisions about their own lives to the full extent of their abilities. Specific performance indicators might include holding monthly tenants' meetings, sending invitations to all, levels of attendance achieved, individual involvement in drawing up and reviewing each care plan and so on. Most of these are easily measurable, although there are degrees of individual involvement and it would be easy for consideration of this to become tokenistic. Indicators might therefore need to be quite robust in what they measure and how they measure it. Again as in research, 'triangulation' of the data (gathering it in several different forms and cross-checking them) may be useful. At the extreme, it may also provide checks and balances against the continuation of any malpractice which one form of monitoring alone has failed to detect.

The above example of tenant participation is fairly straightforward in terms of who is involved in giving and receiving the service. Were the quality of a whole care package to be monitored, however, this might involve several different service providers and some services with a chain of people involved, from suppliers of each foodstuff used in meals on wheels, for example, through the company that prepares the meals, the local authority as purchaser, and the delivery process. There will be contractual arrangements at each stage which can each have standards written in, for example the nutritional content and portion sizes of the completed meals. The outcome of the care provided to the user will depend on all these people getting it right first time, every time. It is important to think quite broadly about this when considering what service people are offered in your setting. In social services offices, for example, the impression people receive can be as influenced by the reception staff as by the duty officer they see. This means not only that users should be given the opportunity to comment on reception services, but also that receptionists should be involved in the discussions that set quality standards and should receive adequate training.

User and carer views

The ultimate test of quality will always be what users and their families think of the services we provide. They are the equivalent of 'customers' in the business world and they have a right to be involved, both in setting standards and reviewing the outcomes of care. It does take special efforts to obtain the views of social work's consumers. There is evidence, for example, that few children in the care system know about complaints procedures, let alone use them (Wallis and Frost, 1998; and see below).

We need to think both about what users are asked to comment on and how this can best be done. Most publications on quality offer broad criteria by which quality can be measured, in terms of user response. Maxwell (1984), for example, lists:

- *appropriateness:* Individuals get the right response to their needs
- *equity:* Individuals and groups get a fair share of the resources available
- *acceptability:* Services satisfy users' expectations
- *accessibility:* Services satisfy requirements such as convenience, openness, information, physical layout and so on
- *efficiency:* Resources are used to generate the maximum benefit for those in need
- *effectiveness:* Services achieve the intended outcomes.

Given that many users have to contribute towards the cost of services, one might add *value for money* to this list. Furthermore, if services are going to be user-friendly, Pfeffer and Coote (1991) add that they should be:

- *participative,* involving service users in decisions and choices
- *integrated* across agencies and sectors of care
- *responsive* to individual needs through flexibility.

Although it is not easy to set standards with users or build these into contracts, increasingly, useful work is being done on this which can be drawn upon. There are, for example, standards for domiciliary services developed through consultation with users. They are: reliability, continuity, kindness and understanding shown to users, cheerfulness and competence, flexibility, and knowledge of the needs and wishes of users (Nuffield Institute for Health and United Kingdom Homecare Association, 1997). Although this work can be transferred from the private to the public sector, it is always going to be more difficult to extend it to informal carers such as neighbours or volunteers, upon whom many users rely. So there will be limits to what can be achieved.

In statutory social work, the standards to be met will need to reflect wider expectations, not just what a service user or their family might want. Even then, Casson and Manning (1997) show how parents' views can be incorporated into child protection standards in, for example, the consistency of the worker, being kept informed at all stages of an investigation, and having an opportunity to comment on the accuracy of reports. Children and young people have also asked for some say over whether and how they are medically examined and the way their suspected abuse is investigated.

Users and carers have also been involved as members of inspection teams, to ensure that the perspectives and experiences of these groups are high up the list of matters considered and discussed in inspections. The Social Services Inspectorate involved 'lay assessors' for a number of years and experimented with the involvement of young people in inspections of children's services (Hibbert, 2003).

Formal standard-setting

Perhaps because there is some difficulty in measuring quality standards in interpersonal fields such as social work, imported frameworks have proved attractive. They have also had the benefit of providing business credibility for social services by drawing a comparison with other sectors of the economy. In the early days of concerns with quality, some social work services sought a British Standards award, BS 5750 Part 2, which set a standard, not for a particular product, but for a quality assurance system and its component procedures. This, in turn, was used as the basis of the ISO 9000 series, first established in 1994.

The BS/ISO approach is essentially a maintenance model and arguably has been largely superseded. A more developed quality management system would go beyond this into taking action, for continual improvement based on the appraisal of actual achievement. The same processes of consultation, and of staff and user involvement, would go into determining action plans and their review as went into setting the initial quality standards.

The Charter Mark scheme for the public sector was launched by central government in the early 1990s, to provide an independently audited judgement on the quality of public services. The scheme was relaunched in 2003, as a lever for change for the whole public sector, recognising organisations that are setting standards based on what the customer wants, offer choice to the customer, promote continuous improvement, and free up frontline staff to carry out their core tasks (http://www.chartermark.gov.uk). The criteria for the award are that the organisation must be seen to:

- set standards and perform well
- engage actively with customers, partners and staff
- be fair and accessible to everyone and promote choice
- continuously develop and improve
- use resources effectively and imaginatively
- contribute to improving opportunities and quality of life in the communities served.

Investors in People (IiP) (http://www.investorsinpeople.co.uk) was launched in 1991 as a government-sponsored quality scheme on the management of people for all sectors. The scheme is now franchised around the world. The government would like all employers to achieve the award and most local authorities and many voluntary and private sector organisations have either done so already or are working towards it. The scheme can sit alongside other schemes, such as EFQM (see below). IiP is based on an independent audit against a number of HRM criteria. Evidence includes surveys of and interviews with staff to test the extent to which they are involved in the business and understand their role in it. An organisation with poor communication with staff and low morale will not achieve the award. Investors in People has also recently relaunched its approach. The judgement is now based on four principles – commitment, planning, action and evaluation – each with a series of indicators and sources of evidence.

While organisations are increasingly volunteering to measure up to one set of standards or another, many in social work and social care find it more relevant to use systems of standards frameworks that are specific to their own employment sector. Hence the National Occupational Standards (NOS) for social care are being adapted by some social services organisations as a wider measure of quality, while the Business Excellence Model (BEM), developed by the European Foundation for Quality Management (EFQM), has updated for the public sector its aim of assessing areas of strength across the organisation as a whole and developing annual improvement plans so as to make the striving for excellence a continuous process (see summary in Darvill, 1998b). A survey of the sector has shown that most SSDs have chosen to apply one formalised set of standards or another, and sometimes more than one (Darvill, 1998b).

National frameworks

At the same time as the public sector has been making its own selection of more rigorous approaches to quality and setting its own quality standards, external checks over which there is no choice have also proliferated. This has been a conscious strategy of central government. Joint Reviews of Local Authority Social Services (www.joint-reviews.gov.uk) originated in the decision to give local authorities lead responsibility for community care budgets, including a substantial transfer of funding from the social security budget and new responsibilities for commissioning services from the private sector. The government established this new review initiative as a joint responsibility of the Audit Commission (which monitors local government performance across the board) and the then Social Services Inspectorate (SSI) of the Department of Health. SSI Wales later became a partner. Joint Reviews provided a comprehensive evaluation of the whole social services function of the local council, covering all but one of the authorities in England and Wales over the seven-year period to 2003. Over that time, a developing methodology sharpened up the criteria for evaluating effectiveness in social services management and delivery, with the intention of creating what has been called a 'no excuses' culture (Hirst, 1998). Reports on the weakest departments attracted significant publicity and some directors were forced to retire early, particularly where authorities were perceived as failing to safeguard children. The Joint Review reports, together with the annual national overview reports, provide a unique insight into the trends in social work and social service management across the whole country at that time (for example DoH/SSI and the Audit Commission, 2002, 2003, or see Joint Reviews, 2004 and http://www.joint-reviews. gov.uk/annrep02.html).

For New Labour, centralised regulation has consistently formed a key element of its drive to reform and modernise public services. Tony Blair stated: 'The role of the centre will be to set a framework of national priorities and then a system of accountability, inspection and intervention to maintain basic standards across the country' (http://www.number-10.gov.uk/output/page257.asp). Although not accompanied by the level of devolution of autonomy to frontline staff that was also promised, this framework has indeed been put in place. First, Best Value Performance Plans (DETR, 1998; and see above) for the whole local authority were required to be inspected by the Audit Commission and other inspectorates, who also had the task of conducting individual service reviews and making a public report on how well the local council was doing.

At around the same time, the Performance Assessment Framework for social services in England was announced in the White Paper *Modernising Social Services*, published in November 1998 (DoH, 1998a). This was a major new initiative, probably the first of its kind in the world, which had a dramatic impact on the management and organisation of services and also on social work practice. It identified a range of indicators for all social services, to be collected in each local authority and collated nationally as a basis for publishing comparative data on the performance of local councils. For the first time, this provided a public statement of targets for social work and social services and a mechanism for measuring how well councils were doing – in effect, the first ever nationally established framework for describing and evaluating the effectiveness of social work. At the same time, it raised significant methodological problems and data collection questions. Many councils have struggled to engage frontline staff in this latter process, leaving people frustrated about the burden of collecting information with no obvious or immediate benefit for staff or service users. Nevertheless, in the best councils (see, for example, DoH/SSI and Audit Commission, 2003, or http://www.joint-reviews.gov.uk/reviews/Kirklees.htm), staff and managers have used the process to engage in a positive process of service improvement.

Not long after, the government announced a wider ranging appoach to evaluating local council performance in the White Paper, *Strong Local Leadership: Quality Public Services* (ODPM, 2001). This introduced a new performance management framework for local government, including social services, intended to deliver 'a balanced and wide ranging assessment of performance against clearly defined priorities' (http://www.odpm.gov.uk/stellent/groups/odpm-localgov/documents/page/odpm_localgov_605183.hcsp). These Comprehensive Performance Assessments (CPAs) brought together, for the first time, an overview of the performance of every council 'to provide a basis for central and local government to work together to achieve improvements in local services' (ibid.). The result of the first CPA was announced by the Audit Commission in December 2002 (see www.councilperformance.gov.uk or www.audit-commission.gov.uk/cpa/index.asp). These assessments integrated a wide range of performance information to deliver an overall judgement based on the delivery of core services and the corporate strength of each council. Councils that did very well (3 star) were awarded 'freedom and flexibilities', including more control over their budgets and an 'inspection holiday'. The 15 most poorly performing councils, according to this exercise, on the other hand were targeted for fast-track improvement, with intervention including additional resources and monitoring.

Over the years, then, the political certainty has been emerging that there can and should be a national agenda as to what is 'good enough'. This underpins everything from the Best Value criteria utilised by local authorities in operating their own services to the national standards now applied in the inspection and registration functions held by the National Commissions for Care Standards (which inspect community services as well as care homes). For the first time, this approach to quality gives users and carers the ability to challenge any authority that falls short of a nationally agreed benchmark. The General Social Care Council (GSCC – in England and the respective Social Care/Services Councils elsewhere in the UK) also has a role in maintaining standards through the registration and discipline of staff.

From the Joint Review overviews, some clear conclusions have emerged about what makes for effective services and what constitutes a poor council (DoH/SSI and the Audit Commission, 2002). The attributes of a successful council, providing good social services, have been shown to include:

● clear strategic direction
● understanding the priorities of local people and how these are changing
● openness to challenge and willingness to change direction
● clear roles and responsibilities between councillors and officers
● willingness to share control and resources with other agencies
● ambition to raise the standards of core services
● decision-making on the basis of good information

- using resources to good effect, levering change and achieving best value
- cascading objectives through the organisation and monitoring progress (ibid.).

Some of the key findings point to the importance of getting the basics right (DoH/SSI and the Audit Commission, 2002). User satisfaction seems related to a speedy and personal response and a trusting relationship with a social worker or key worker, often more so than to amounts of money spent on services. Core services matter more to people than the distractions of new initiatives and high-profile projects. Developing the skills of staff and ensuring good management of core tasks pays off in better services.

So, while a local authority remains responsible for judging its own performance, increasingly this is required to take place against national standards. Within this, the local authority is free to measure its services against its own published eligibility criteria for assessment and receipt of services.

The performance agenda is not without its critics (see Hunter and Blackmore, 2003, for a useful summary). The sheer bureaucracy and cost involved are contentious, particularly as they tend to compete with getting on with the job. There are notorious difficulties associated with knowing what to measure and how to measure it, and once the measures and mechanisms have been decided, they may be manipulated by clever councils. The limited number of gradings (0–3 stars) creates a broadbrush impression and lumps together those who just missed a higher ranking with those who narrowly avoided a lower one. Once the results are published, possibly undue attention is paid to 'failing' councils and poorly performing teams, when improvement may actually be needed across the board or could be more usefully focused elsewhere. Above all, the exercise makes it appear that everything is under local councils' control, whereas many would argue that shortfalls in central government funding outweigh most other causes of difficulty. Meanwhile, theoreticians increasingly take the view that searching for linear cause and effect of any kind in complex public services is illusory (Haynes, 2003).

In the voluntary sector, there is less imposition of standards from above. A 'compact' aims to deliver certain pledges from government on respecting the sector's independence and right to longer term funding in return for an undertaking by voluntary organisations themselves. They are expected to promote best practice and equality of opportunity, and to consult and involve users wherever possible, including in the development and management of activities and services (Hunter, 1999). This is the nearest government can get to imposing standards on a sector over which it has no direct control beyond the broadest considerations of financial rectitude and non-political activity. It is a recognition that the 'third sector' plays an increasing role in the direct delivery of social care services, is a major player in the economy of the UK, with over 6 per cent of national employment and almost as many again engaged in volunteer activities (Kendall with Almond, 1998), and that government cannot deliver its policies without a high quality contribution from this source.

Quality systems

Quality management requires a 'disciplined and systematic approach' (Warr and Kelly, 1992, p. 2). The most basic action to improve quality – measuring outcomes, taking feedback and using these in future planning – returns us to the input/output/throughput systems feedback loop we saw in Chapter 2.

It is not always necessary for the impetus to come from senior management. It is perfectly possible to introduce a quality assurance system at team or establishment level and models for doing so can even be bought off the peg. Grover (1992) describes how a multidisciplinary mental health project brought in a consultant to help them review their systems of staffing and finance, linking with external agencies, team functioning and service delivery. A constantly repeating quality cycle of action, monitoring and change was introduced, with detailed action points. The staff jointly owned the process of change, although service users' views were not fully integrated. Although not perfect, this is a good example of a small group of practitioners in a community care setting taking a systems approach to change without waiting for their parent agencies at the macro-level to do it all for them.

Quality circles

One particular technique imported from Japan which emphasised the involvement of staff lower down the hierarchy was *quality circles*. The idea was to move away from rigid management hierarchies and compartmentalisation of task performance and to encourage groups of employees to meet with a facilitator to solve problems affecting everyone in relation to the product or working conditions. Members of quality circles would be offered training in problem definition and analysis, teamwork and communication. Their involvement, personal growth and increased job satisfaction were said to be good for corporate success. In the UK, employees were mainly indifferent or hostile to quality circles and there has also been scepticism as to what kinds of problems they were ever really engaged in solving and how useful an approach can be if it is a technical 'bolt-on' to an otherwise unchanged organisation (McKenna and Beech, 1995).

Total quality management (TQM)

TQM (Piggott and Piggott, 1992; see also Morgan and Murgatroyd, 1994 for a public sector application) attempts to go beyond quality systems into a culture of quality for the whole organisation. Consequently, it combines both quality control and quality assurance. It emphasises top-down vision and planning, including commitment to quality at the most senior level, and bottom-up involvement and motivation of all the staff. It is strategically driven, in terms of 'hard' factors such as performance standards and the monitoring of quantitative management information (numbers of users, cost of services, outcomes of interventions), and particularly because it operates within corporate objectives, but it also emphasises 'soft', people-oriented factors such as customer care, staff skills and teamwork. The hallmarks of the approach are *getting things right first time every time,* ending up with customers who are delighted rather than merely satisfied, and continually improving performance (see Chapter 6 on ways of building this in through appraisal and staff development). Casson and Manning (1997) point out that it implies implementing a system sufficiently robust to meet all the agreed standards even when people go on leave or there are temporary staff employed. This includes guidelines detailed enough to remind the child protection social worker to check that the room is at a comfortable temperature and that there are tissues handy before every case conference. It is the implementation that counts, however: 'Every specification of quality must have clearly thought out ways of consistently delivering it' (Casson and Manning, 1997, p. 28). This presents a significant challenge to those organisations that are reliant on a changing procession of agency staff just to keep the door open.

As its name suggests, TQM cannot be envisaged as an add-on, but typically requires a *pervasive culture change* towards a management approach that values every member of the organisation. Quality is the key to success and it is the responsibility of every employee. As a result, both staff development and staff care become important (see Chapter 6). TQM also needs all parts of the organisation to be working well together and it needs action rather than rhetoric.

Often, the strategy is seen as needing to start by making staff feel involved and motivated, 'winning their hearts and minds', before working outwards to service users and carers. The views and efforts of staff become as important as management-led or external regulation, monitoring and inspection. Importantly, this means the whole staff group being involved, not devolving all the responsibility for quality to individual staff (although there will, of course, be designated staff to operate the quality system). Similarly, if Ellis and Whittington's (1998) idea of a quality assurance group is taken up, those who have been interested in joining the group will have to make special efforts to ensure that everyone else remains committed. It might be easier to involve a whole team or staff group in taking quality on board, even if particular tasks are delegated and reported back on as the work progresses. It is empowering for staff to be accorded this kind of dignity and respect, and to be thought capable of innovative ideas, not just of carrying out tasks in a routine way to meet targets they had no part in setting. This has to have constant support from the very top so that everyone sees quality as part of the job they are expected to do. Staff also have to feel trusted before they will, in turn, feel committed.

TQM is closely linked with HRM because it brings to the fore all the various staffing issues (McKenna and Beech, 1995). In particular, staff development becomes doubly important because it not only improves performance but may become the major channel for quality issues. One would also expect to see flexibility in working practices, autonomy in decision-making and a supportive environment for staff in any organisation committed to TQM. How far this is possible when corporate objectives remain the guiding force (in other words, what would really happen if a team stepped out of line or had a totally off-beam idea) is questionable. But, in some social work agencies, even a degree of change in this direction might be very much valued by staff.

In social work, an easy-to-follow guide is available for any manager seeking to emulate the approach (Casson and Manning, 1997) and there is also a quality assurance workbook available for social care settings (Ellis and Whittington, 1998). Both publications include learning objectives, exercises, activities and practice examples. They could be used by individuals studying for an award, or by a whole team or a social work agency proposing to implement change along quality-inspired lines.

The practitioner as quality manager

As we discussed in Chapter 1, there is scope to regard every practitioner as a manager. In so far as the individual care manager has the responsibility for the 'total quality of care as it is experienced by the user' (DoH/SSI and the Scottish Office Social Work Services Group, 1991, para. 6.13), this is certainly true of quality standards. In monitoring the effective working of the individual care plan, for example, a care manager may be responsible not only for his or her own work but for enforcing the standards specified in contracts with contributors to the plan and overseeing any agreements with carers or volunteers. The concept of 'service congruence' covers the broader question of whether the care plan as a whole is achieving what it set out to achieve. The care manager will need to create his or her own systems for feedback as well as identifying measures of success. The satisfaction of the user will, of course, be of primary importance. For some complex plans where the user is, for example, confused and unable to give direct feedback, a similar range of views may need to be sought as were involved in the original assessment of need. In such a case, the carer's views are likely to assume a major role.

Critique of quality in social care

Various criticisms have been levelled against ideas of quality management as they operate in social work. These are:

● *Unsuitability*: The pursuit of quality was brought into social work and social care from the industrial and commercial world, and there is both an upside and a downside to this. On the one hand, it makes even greater sense to aim for high standards when you are working directly with people rather than manufacturing washing machine parts or selling clothes, because improvements in quality will lead to an improved quality of life at the most basic level. On the other hand, it makes results harder to judge, since you cannot physically measure a product or count sales or profits when your job is caring for people in a residential home. Of course, the occupancy rate of the home and the balancing of the budget are important, but they are not the whole story. Standards and performance indicators can be set, but they will always be imprecise, involving value-based and sometimes essentially political judgements as to what constitutes an improvement.

- *Political issues*: A local authority's own recording of unmet need, while raising legal complexities (because there are limitations on the extent to which an authority's lack of resources can be taken into account when deciding whether or not to provide services; see Paterson, 1999, pp. 153–4), could potentially act as one of the most important mechanisms for feeding into future planning, leading to improved or better targeted services. Most quality systems work by checking standards against a predetermined norm. It is particularly difficult to take issue with this and to argue that the norm itself is wrong, either in principle (top-down services, for example) or in operation (for example over-narrow eligibility criteria).
- *Proliferating bueaucracy*: We are moving into an era where there is a risk of duplication in monitoring quality. Money that might otherwise have gone into providing direct services is being channelled into more and more bureaucracy surrounding checking up on provision. In addition to the cost to users and carers in reduced spending on services, this may make staff feel that they are under surveillance rather than involved in a quality culture.
- *User empowerment and anti-oppressive practice*: The extent to which anti-oppressive objectives are integrated into thinking about quality, or the voice of service users and carers built into monitoring and other quality systems, varies greatly. Quality models are no exception to the fact that most management literature comes from the conservative ethos of business administration. Social work thinking about anti-oppressive practice and user empowerment gives us our own ways of approaching many of the issues in question but, up to now,

social work managers (many of whom take MBAs with little public sector, let alone social work content) have often failed to respond to this more radical challenge. As we saw above, Adams' (1998) quality maximisation model represents one attempt to do so.

Since quality can be judged from a number of viewpoints, it is important to be clear about who is the most important arbiter of quality and who owns the quality measures and outcomes being used. Black groups, for example, have long argued that there can be no quality without equality. Power differentials between the parties – for example between a black woman carer and a white male care manager – should not be ignored when seeking and evaluating feedback on services. This is no doubt one reason why children do not use complaints procedures, although they place unmanageable demand on the anonymous and child-centred services of ChildLine (Wallis and Frost, 1998). Most writing and talk about quality betray their origins in white, male managerialist thinking and leave us still with a long road to travel on equality.

There are links with staff care policies (see Chapter 6), since these should underpin total quality. It took a recruitment and retention crisis to generate interest in funded daycare schemes for those with young children and in responsibility leave for parents and those caring for other relatives, and these are still by no means uniformly available. Yet it is hard to give the best service to users when you are under unreasonable stress yourself in your own working environment.

Concluding thoughts on quality

However it is pursued, quality should give a sense of a continuous process of organisational development, through building on current good practice and making improvements where these are needed. Quality control and quality assurance need not be in conflict and, indeed, many social care agencies are pursuing a mixture of these measures, some at the government's behest and others of their own volition, within an overall ethos of 'customer care'. This is marked by maximising opportunities to obtain user feedback, whether through consultation procedures such as focus groups and local meetings that feed into community care and children's services plans, or more bureaucratic measures such as complaints procedures and monitoring the extent to which quality specifications have been met in service contracts. Staff voices should be heard too, so that they have the chance to raise concerns and make complaints rather than 'blowing the whistle' externally. Indeed, professional organisations in social work, such as the British Association of Social Workers (BASW), were highly concerned with the quality of services offered, long before such matters reached the jargon of management practice. Ironically, in the managerialist era, quality agendas have sometimes tended to rebound on the work-force, with performance measurement used to discipline professionals into conformity (Clarke and Newman, 1997).

Whatever kind of organisation you work for, whether it is a local authority or a health and social services trust, or a voluntary or private agency, it would be interesting to look back over what changes have been adopted in the pursuit of quality. Where has the impetus for change come from? Has it been new legislation or government policy, senior managers going on courses, the fact that others were doing it, a desire to raise the public profile or improve the corporate image, or a dissatisfaction with past performance? Whichever of these has played the greatest role, it is also worth asking yourself to what extent quality thinking has also meant equality thinking, or whether wider social work concerns with the empowerment of disadvantaged user groups and employees have been skated over in the pursuit of a glossy new corporate image.

Whatever the motivation, however, and whatever the eventual outcome, pursuing quality standards inevitably involves processes of change. Rather than wait for change to overtake us, organisational thinking urges us to plan for and manage change so that we can maximise its benefits and minimise its risks.

Managing change

Stable and static organisations concentrate on efficiency and tend to be centralised and bureaucratic as a result (Mintzberg, 1989), along the lines we saw in Chapter 2. As organisations become more complex, however, and as the prevailing conditions within which they operate combine increased expectations with less support, there is a tendency to decentralise and become more organic, developing and adapting as needed in order to manage fragmenting demand and technological advance within a turbulent environment.

Throughout the 1960s and 1970s, as the personal social services grew, they continued to operate as centralised bureaucracies. More recently, social and political pressures have necessitated the appearance of new organisational forms (to encompass the purchaser–provider split in community care, for example), and restructuring has become the hallmark of the age. Staff are also expected to be multiskilled and adaptable, moving about within the organisation or perhaps having serial careers. How do organisations manage these processes of change?

Resistance to change

As early as 1541, Machiavelli (see 1961 edn) noted that anyone attempting innovation had a hard time of it. Those who had done well out of the old ways of working would oppose change on principle, while even those who could see they might do better would be cautious about trying anything new and untested. Consequently, there would be fierce opposition from some and only lukewarm support from others, the latter's support being further dampened by other people's anger or indifference. Machiavelli went on to distinguish between those who could force through changes on their own and those who required the support of others. Although some new directors may act like new brooms sweeping clean and pushing through their favoured reorganisations (albeit without using the physical force that Machiavelli had in mind), it is usually the case in social work that we do need to work out who our allies are, and win over at least some of the opposition, before attempting to steer any major change through a meeting or committee.

Some four centuries later, this need for clarity about who (or what) favours change and who stands in its way was portrayed by Kurt Lewin (1951) in his idea of *force field analysis*. This is a practical approach which assists in the diagnosis of change possibilities. A diagram is constructed which depicts 'driving forces' (those which work for change) and 'restraining forces' (those against change). The method can be used to decide which kind of change is going to be advisable or possible, or as an action tool for carrying through a change which some support and others oppose. Armed with this, the manager can make the necessary decisions about how to cope with innovation and the kind of conflict it may reveal, for example where there are clashes of values or power bases (see Figure 3.1).

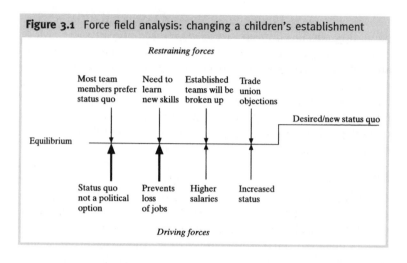

Figure 3.1 Force field analysis: changing a children's establishment

Restraining forces

Most team members prefer status quo

Need to learn new skills

Established teams will be broken up

Trade union objections

Desired/new status quo

Equilibrium

Status quo not a political option

Prevents loss of jobs

Higher salaries

Increased status

Driving forces

Looking at Figure 3.1, it would seem that the fact of accepting change as the only way to stay in a job is going to be a strong motivating factor. So, similar numbers of driving and restraining forces do not necessarily represent equally balanced situations. This can be represented diagrammatically by making some of the arrows thicker than others. The nature of trade union objections will need to be explored and a process of negotiation begun. It may well be that the proposal can be implemented in a way that is as fair as possible to staff while also meeting the new service need that the organisation has identified. Those employees who do not want to learn new skills or weather changes to working conditions may perhaps be given every assistance to find jobs elsewhere. Overall, Figure 3.1 makes it clear that the old equilibrium, the old status quo, will go and that a new one will be established in a different place.

Above all, the analysis reveals that there are two ways to make the change happen: strengthening the support and reducing the opposition. Interestingly, we can have a tendency in debate to concentrate on arguing against those who speak out against us and forget about winning over and working with the potential allies. It is actually a good idea never to go into a meeting to raise a tricky problem or propose a change without having done a rough calculation in advance, on the basis of sounding people out, as to where your support is going to lie and what objections you are going to have to answer. Some of the missing aspects in this model include silent opposition and genuine indifference. Only the protracted debate that real change is likely to involve can bring these into the equation and it should not be supposed from the force field analogy that change is ever a 'one-off' event. It is always a process over time.

Resistance to change is not intrinsically bad (Thompson, 2003). It can hold up ill-advised plans until they have been subjected to more detailed consideration and it can offer some stability where organisations opt for change for its own sake. Employees' natural caution also reminds us that they have a right to know where they stand in terms of job security, terms and conditions of employment and working relationships they may have been building up over a period of years. But there is a *feelings level* as well as a rational level to people's reactions to change. People feel comfortable with familiar ideas, values and working methods; any process of change, according to Lewin (1951), requires them to unfreeze, change, then refreeze into the new arrangements. Good HRM involves giving people enough time to make this adaptation and keeping them well informed as to why change is necessary and what its implications will be, for them and the organisation.

Change techniques

Although we began this exploration of change with a consideration of resistance to it, the management literature is equally full of positive accounts of how people can be innovatory and how they can carry through their ideas for change. Kanter (1991) combines descriptions of how particular individuals are especially good at seeing things in new ways and communicating their visions (requiring, also, the personal qualities of leadership and persistence to see change through), with an awareness that change in modern organisations requires the building of coalitions and teams so that shared effort is rewarded by shared credit.

Thus, interest has moved to the process of change and how this can be managed. It is not about top-down ideas that are imposed by managerial will. Kotter and Schlesinger (1979) identified the following six styles of change management (which are actually ways of overcoming resistance):

- education and communication
- participation and involvement

- facilitation and support
- negotiation and agreement
- manipulation and co-optation
- explicit and implicit coercion.

Negotiation and agreement are generally required when codes and conditions of employment are affected. Participation and involvement are helpful when those with responsibility for implementing change lack the knowledge, power or expertise to do so alone, for example when new computerised systems are introduced. They may also be the favoured style of change within some teams or agencies. Facilitation and support will assist staff to adjust to change and should be routinely available whatever other measures are employed. Change, and the uncertainty it engenders, can be unsettling for staff and a good staff care policy should allow for this, in providing a range of services including financial and pre-retirement planning as well as counselling. Staff may also wish to seek confidential career planning advice if they think their job may be at risk.

Unless we are able to change ourselves, we will have difficulties in effecting change in organisations (Pugh, 1993). The process of implementing change is dynamic; a rigid or unreflexive approach (that is, one where we are unable to see our own part in what is happening) creates fresh resistances in others and new obstacles in operating systems.

While it is true that public sector organisations have faced widespread change in recent years, change is not a constant feature in any single dimension – new priorities coexist with attributes, practices, cultures and systems which have shown a remarkable capacity for endurance. For example, the personal services delivered to service users often remain the same over long periods, even while the arrangements for their management and allocation vary. This has certainly been true of community care, where the fundamental organisational change required to implement the division of service purchasing from service provision was often not accompanied by the intended shift into greater diversity in the services themselves – in the types and timing of meals delivered to people's homes, for example. Sometimes this was due to a sheer lack of innovation and sometimes to conscious opposition, for example in the form of attempts to safeguard the public provision of labour-intensive and hence higher cost services. The apparently slow pace of change has been a source of frustration for government and service users alike, while, conversely, some staff complain that they are sinking in constant change. This begs the question of the best way to implement rapid and sustainable service improvements.

The degree to which change is top-down or bottom-up varies between organisations, according to the distribution of power and the management style adopted. There are examples of change which have arisen from the demands or influence of frontline staff. The development of diversity policies, units and projects in some organisations are examples of this. Eventually, new developments become part of the organisational structures and systems but, at first, there is a struggle to gain support from an unequal power base. Work in a London borough to promote equality of opportunity for women, for example, explicitly used the organisational processes and politics which can at times constitute the barriers to change to achieve the desired results. Notably, a broader women's agenda was recast in terms of the representation of women in senior positions, which brought on board a number of key departments (Itzin, 1995).

Because he recognised that change is threatening, Pugh (1993, pp. 110–12) devised a number of 'rules' for the successful implementation of change in organisations:

- Work hard at establishing the *need for change*.
- Don't only think out the change, *think through it*.
- Initiate change through *informal discussion* to get feedback and participation.
- Positively encourage those concerned to give their *objections*.
- Be prepared to *change yourself* (including by recognising that improvements are possible to any idea and by being open to bottom-up suggestions).
- Monitor the change and *reinforce* it (including telling everyone about the ways in which improvements are being demonstrated).

Change in organisations is likely to happen rapidly only in a situation of crisis. Most changes occur over a long period and usually over a much longer timescale than the change agents had hoped. Studies of councils and departments on special measures, which are consequently receiving considerable support to change quickly, suggest that culture change is likely to take three to four years and, even then, it will not be embedded, although the start of improvement must involve significant frontline service changes that can be implemented in a matter of weeks (NISW, 2001). Given the need to engage others in the process (middle managers often being particularly important to win over) and manage opposition in constructive and helpful ways if the change is to be successfully achieved, considerable time will need to be allowed for the process. Change itself can be debilitating to the individual. Performance and self-esteem can plummet and will not return to normal until those undergoing the change have adapted to it. This may occur in a 'cycle of coping', which includes the stages of denial, defence, discarding (when it is realised that change is inevitable), adaptation and finally internalisation (Carnall, 1995). Change agents can anticipate this cycle, learning from the early stages about issues that may need to be tackled before the change will work and giving staff every support to move through to the point where they can incorporate the changes into their ways of working.

Involving staff in change

A project devised by those affected will often produce less resistance. Where staff see that the change reduces rather than increases their burdens, they are more likely to welcome it and, if autonomy and professional values are not threatened, acceptance will probably be gained. It is critical, therefore, that a team is involved and consulted and that a consensus on the decision is attempted. Moreover, a plan which has built-in revision and reconsideration conveys empathy to opponents who need to have their objections taken seriously. Where there is defensiveness, frequently there is underlying fear; again, the manager who listens, gives clear information and can be trusted is more likely to negotiate needed changes successfully.

Of course, not all ideas for change come from the top. Indeed, it could be argued that the most novel ones emerge away from those in power who may well see innovation as a disturbance. Team leaders, for example, can cash in on times of change and organisational crisis to push forward their own plans, which may be more likely to be adopted at moments when solutions are actively being sought. There are also certain environments that favour the involvement of staff in change. Factors which can help include: decentralised structures with open channels of communication; well resourced teams with time to discuss ideas; clear procedures from which to start; a risk-taking ethos; and staff who enjoy their work and are committed to getting it right.

Nonetheless, initiating change in social welfare is especially difficult because of the interdependent nature of organisations with other systems. For example, say a voluntary body decided to implement a team approach to resource allocation. It might emerge that others, such as the purchasers of services, other funders or the Charity Commission, required one nominated individual to hold responsibility. In such a circumstance, management tactics might be to foster 'facilitative interdependence' (Weiner, 1982, p. 115) by:

● identifying interagency needs and issues and ensuring that the planned change would contribute to service improvement
● promoting the visibility of the change and reinforcing its positive ramifications for all the services
● forging links with other bodies, explaining the reasons for change, while lobbying for support from other systems in the task environment and other networks so that there would be a greater chance of collaboration and coordination.

Whatever the dynamics of change, if the results of introducing new ideas are counterintuitive, having less than the desired effect, this can be traced back to improper or incomplete planning (Luciano, 1979). The systems view of organisations, as presented in Chapter 2, saw them as having their own internal subsystems and being part of a super-system. If there are planned changes, a proper outcome could result from estimating the implications for the subsystems and external systems with which the organisation interrelates. The growing interdependency of the personal social services and the health services, especially, will encourage jointly planned and executed projects which will need to manage the complexities as well as the possibilities for change across organisational boundaries.

One management technique which can prove useful when change becomes necessary is MBWA or 'management by walking [or wandering] about'. Peters and Waterman (1982), although not the originators of this idea, did draw attention to its value. The most senior manager, in particular, will gain trust and respect by becoming a recognisable face to employees and asking their opinions.

Equally importantly, he or she will have a sense of what is happening at the 'front line', will be able to forestall many problems, and will be much better able to anticipate the need for change and win agreement to it.

The only way to be genuinely well informed is to meet all levels of employees at their workplace. This is also an excellent way of raising morale and demonstrating a shared commitment to improving the quality of service the organisation offers. The manager becomes more visible and can also more effectively lead by example if he or she is not permanently shut in an executive office behind a large desk. MBWA is not just about asking the royal walkabout question: 'And what do you do?' It can be targeted on getting to know who are the key troubleshooters in the different locations and forging links with them, checking that people are committed to the overall aims and values of the organisation, finding out how work is organised on the ground, looking for ways to make links and minimise conflicts across the organisation (because the manager has this oversight better than anybody), and finding out what will motivate or free people up to do a better job (Leigh, 1988, p. 187). More precisely, the visit can be made to discuss the organisation's mission statement or talk through a particular process of change. It is important to ensure that MBWA does not make people feel they are being inspected or give line managers any reason to think their authority is being undermined. The overall aim is to create a climate of openness and it may be particularly positive if teams, establishments or projects feel able to invite managers in when they have something new or positive to share. In social work, managers may be required to make rota visits to establishments for which they are responsible. Although these do have a more formal, managerial function, it may still be possible to inject them with some of the positives of MBWA by adopting an open manner and focusing on some of the same issues.

Although MBWA can help to change an organisation, it focuses only on what the people at the top do. In order to change a whole organisational culture, something more thoroughgoing will be needed. TQM is one such approach. McKenna and Beech (1995, citing Schein, 1985) point to a number of ways in which HRM issues pervading a whole organisation can combine with leadership style to change the culture. Leaders are important *role models* – they can set an example through the issues they focus on, the way they react to crises, and by enabling others to develop as future managers in a supportive environment. The whole organisation, however, also sends important messages through what it values in selecting, rewarding and promoting staff, what it emphasises in policy-making (in everything from staff development to restructuring), through its physical environment (pleasant reception areas, multilingual sign-boards) and corporate imagery (coat of arms, logo), its formal mission and customer care statements and the informal mythology to which it gives rise. Most of these can be manipulated and it is not impossible to inaugurate a new era with a new message.

Unfortunately, cultures of stress, blame, managerialism and competition are not usually chosen but come about through a combination of wider welfare changes, public image and pressure of work. Changing such an ethos is not easy but it may well be necessary if staff are not only to survive but also give a high quality service. Thompson et al. (1996, p. 662) urge 'an explicit strategy of culture change' in the face of evidence that organisations themselves can both engender and allay stress (see also DoH/SSI and the Audit Commission, 2002).

Change in social work

Rather than focusing always on staff as the cause of problems, cutting-edge thinking in social work now sees the whole agency as needing to become a 'learning organisation' (originally Argyris and Schön, 1978, now in wider use – notably, see Senge, 1990) and a 'competent workplace' (Pottage and Evans, 1994), a term which implies harnessing the practice wisdom and skills of the workforce within the overall mission of the agency to give the most effective response to users. It is the culture of the workplace that brings out the best in staff and even the best of workers and teams will become demoralised in a poorly managed organisation.

There is a literature specifically aimed at social work profession-als and managers who seek planned change within their own organisations (NISW, 1995; Smale, 1996, 1997; and Gann, 1996 for the voluntary sector; see also Rosen, 1999). Indeed, social work has its own model of managing change available in the form of a workbook (Smale, 1996). Its message involves breaking down the process into clearly defined components. It also places considerable stress on the 'people' aspects of change. Before action even begins, it is considered important:

- to plan it with all the people involved
- to share the problem with them so that they become part of finding the solution and making it work
- to identify the significant people and connections for the particular changes that will then be needed
- to see managing the process of change as one of working with the people involved
- to recognise that all new ways of working, new technology and new policies have change implications of some magnitude for staff.

Smale (1996) puts the emphasis on the people involved and, within this, he encompasses such skills as: enabling, persuading, reassuring, bargaining, forming alliances and partnerships, on the one hand, and, where necessary, avoiding, bypassing or seeing one's own ideas carry the day, on the other. Smale also personalises the forces for and against change by asking questions such as who wants change and why, who finds the status quo to be a problem, how people's circumstances could be improved by implementing change, and what can stay the same so that people do not suffer unnecessary loss or unintended consequences. He also asks what behaviours and relationships will need to alter as a result of the innovation, and recognises that it is easier to adapt to new tasks than to changes in the way we relate to other people. He looks for what the proposed change means to people, including in terms of clashes of values and symbolic meanings. He looks for the enthusiasts and those who will be motivated by the change, and he breaks down the key players into a number of roles, from 'innovators' who introduce the idea and 'product champions' who spread the word, through 'change agents', with their 'process consultants' on the outside and 'minders' in senior management, to active 'opponents' and 'laggards' who prefer to live in the past. Nor is this picture individualised, as the list also includes 'opinion leaders' and 'network entrepreneurs', for example.

The Smale model is an action-oriented one, with steps through the process and questions to ask oneself at each point. Again, there is both a 'people' feel and a sense of the force field analysis throughout, with tips on which types and groups of people to bring together or support to make the change happen, which to regard as crucial in terms of consent or resources, and which to keep out of the way because they could block the change or take counteraction. There are other ways, too, in which the social work roots of the model are clear, for example recognising that people need to mourn what they experience as losses, that people know their own jobs and consequently what deadlines are realistic for them, that there will be staff development dimensions of any change and a need for managers to exchange information, and that there may need to be new team-building opportunities or attention to interdisciplinary working. Finally, he follows through into feedback after the change and continues to show the force field influence by suggesting that working with allies at this stage may give a better return than concentrating on overcoming resistance. It may also be more effective to look at what underlies the resistance and whether this indicates that modifications are needed to the process or nature of the change. Smale also gives the good advice that subsequent evaluation needs to look not solely at how smoothly the process went, but also at whether the original problem has been solved and whether any new ones have been created that may require further problem-solving and change efforts.

Following a people-oriented model like Smale's should help to prevent too many casualties of change. In social work, after all, people are often not being entirely self-interested in opposing change. They may have the interests of users and carers at heart and sincerely believe that a poorer service will result. Perhaps the move towards greater consultation with users and local communities, under the Best Value initiative for example, can help to avoid confrontation between opposing groups within organisations who all think they know best.

Organisational contexts

The organisational context is also important. While some organisations are actively empowering, most show some resistance to change:

> Some agencies are hospitable to empowerment as a goal. Others are not. Some don't know because they have never faced a situation which challenged their values to any serious degree. Agency culture grows over time, often starting with a very positive philosophy about human dignity and meeting needs. Then, under the accretions of paper work, over-worked

> staff, ill-tempers, rigid conformity to rules – to say nothing
> of difficult clientele and intractable problems, policies begin
> to change – both formal and informal ones – and the clients
> begin to receive a disservice . . . For many reasons, clients
> can find themselves feeling utterly frustrated and helpless in
> dealing with an agency whose mission is ostensibly to serve
> them.
> (Pernell, 1986, p. 112)

Many are skilled at absorbing and diluting new ideas in accord
with their own norms, demanding compromises and spinning out
decisions until momentum is lost (Cohen, 1975, p. 92). As Stock
Whitaker (1975, p. 426) points out, 'covert resistance' – verbal
assurances without active support – can be far harder to deal with
than out-and-out opposition because it may emerge only gradually
and be quite subtle in its manifestations. She gives the example of
an agency where key powerful personnel absented themselves from
staff meetings, thus rendering an external facilitator impotent to
effect change.

It is certainly well worth putting together a good case to
persuade management of what your ideas have to offer and how
they can be used in a particular instance. To second-guess the
response with the untested plea, 'management would *never* let us
try that here', is certainly never justified, since there is frequently
more space in which to operate than is assumed and, even where
there is not, it is morally more acceptable to look, and if necessary
campaign, for more freedom of activity than to collude with its
absence. As Pernell (1986, p. 112), drawing on work on black
empowerment, has said of any agency's service delivery system:

> The importance and potential that it might be changed from
> obstacle course to opportunity system requires of workers
> who identify the need for change a search for their own
> powers of persuasiveness, of diplomatic skill, of assessment
> of accessibility and leverage points for inducing modification
> of current practices.

Other agencies beyond one's own employer, such as funders and
contractors, can also present obstacles. Similar skills are needed for
working with them.

An organisation that copes well with change can certainly be thought of as a learning organisation – an organisation that helps people to learn by constantly questioning itself (Argyris and Schön, 1978). If people continually have to adjust their behaviour to fit the pre-existing norms of the organisation when they take decisions in its name, whatever the outside evidence of a need for the organisation itself to change, there is no real learning – and no amount of quality control or quality audit will challenge this because the monitoring assumes that the standards and procedures are all correct. Only when the organisation as a whole questions its norms, in the face of a conflict of values, does it restructure its strategies and assumptions (which also govern its employees' behaviour) in a healthy new way. When it does this, it not only learns, but learns to learn again in the future. When it fails to learn new lessons, it perpetuates conflict and encourages entrenched positions. Aryris and Schön call the two reactions 'single-loop' and 'double-loop' learning, double-loop being the one that feeds back in to create change for the future.

As will be familiar from Schön's other work on 'reflective practice', he and Argyris believe that it is only as managers (and professionals) examine their own reasoning processes that they will understand how they respond to the errors, mismatches and conflicts that present the prime opportunities for new learning, and, crucially (for people involved in practice learning as much as managers), how they help others to do this. There are similar concepts in groupwork practice and crisis theory, which suggest that it is at times of difficulty that groups and individuals have the greatest energy and opportunity to move forward in new ways. We will also see in Chapters 5 and 6 how encouraging people to talk about such key points can be used in selection and appraisal interviews.

Examples of social work organisations altering their norms in recent years in the face of new values from outside have been the adoption (partially at least) of a social model of disability and hugely altered attitudes towards the rights of people with learning difficulties to live an independent and fulfilling life. Previously, the talk was all of disabled people 'adjusting' to their limitations, not of society (including social work) adjusting the way it treated them.

Change is possible, then, but to manage it rather than be bowled over by it requires vision, persistence and strong alliances. The most effective of these are undoubtedly where staff and local people can pursue shared objectives.

Conclusion

This chapter has been bound together by a sense of forward movement – towards the pursuit of both the highest quality and of managed change to attain that goal. Nothing in the organisational world stays still nowadays and there is a real feeling of needing to take hold of what is happening before it takes hold of us. Considerations of quality standards and managed change demonstrate that there is a role for staff at every level in thinking through and working towards the delivery of the best outcomes for service users and their carers. From this sense of a shared endeavour throughout the organisation, we will now move on to look at the role of top managers in offering leadership and a management vision. Far from cutting across the views of others, effective leadership should help everyone else to feel that they are playing a vital part in crewing a ship that is being competently steered through ever choppier waters. Chapter 4 will go beyond that, however, to look at the greater caution introduced by complexity theory, which suggests that even the best managers are coping with unpredictability rather than rational decision-making and, consequently, it is flexibility and creativity that will win out over certainty and direction.

4 | Management as vision, strategy and leadership, or management of uncertainty?

Although providing leadership is only one aspect of what the top manager does, it is the most visible – particularly when it is lacking. In the view of the project director for the Audit Commission/Social Services Inspectorate Joint Reviews: 'Where authorities are failing, it's usually down to a lack of a clear steer and grip on the organisation by management and a lack of accountability' (Hirst, 1998, p. 8). He also relates this to the overall culture of an organisation, as we did in Chapter 3. In a later report, the Joint Review Team interviewed directors in departments that had implemented successful changes and was 'struck by how often questions about the critical success factors led directors to reflect not only on their actions, but also on their style and approach' (DoH/SSI and the Audit Commission, 2002). Consequently, leadership is often seen as a key element of management. To show how it relates to the whole organisation, we link it to vision and strategy and go on to comment on leadership roles and styles.

It is often asked whether leaders are born or made. Whatever the factors that create inspirational leaders, the skills they employ can be learned and developed. All managers can develop their ability to motivate staff and manage operations.

Vision and mission: the link with strategic planning

When we are going about our day-to-day work, we have little time to stop and think about the wider purposes we are serving or whether all our efforts are being expended to good effect. For the senior manager, this is an essential part of the job. Like driving a car, managing an organisation is more than operating technical controls; you have to know where you want to go and steer the whole vehicle accordingly, even in the face of traffic that is trying to cut right across your path.

In social change work, it can be rewarding to pause and ask the big questions: What is the vision of the world we are trying to create? What style of organisation would be best at achieving this? The best motivators and innovators have a clear image of where they are trying to get and are extremely good at taking other people with them.

Vision refers to hopes and aspirations for the organisation over the longer term, usually involving an explicit value base. It should ideally be developed with staff and stakeholders and be recognised and supported by them all. A vision must always be positive. A book on opposing homophobia presents the example of imagining a world without sex-role stereotypes, revealing the extent to which violence, the expression of affection, life ambitions, the placing of love and trust in other people, the choice of careers and personal appearance, and many other fundamental aspects of human life revolve around narrow ideas of sexual identity (Pharr, 1988). There are unquestioned assumptions of equivalent magnitude operating in organisations, often serving to maintain the status quo, which it takes vision to open up to scrutiny. The feminisation of management thinking is one example of questioning the old order, as we shall see in Chapter 7.

In social work and social care, it takes managers with vision to bring the customer care and staff care agendas to the centre of attention. It also takes vision to shift managerial concerns beyond narrow conceptions of balanced budgets and procedural conformity onto quality standards that reflect the aspirations of all the interested parties, including service users and their families, for whom the best outcomes of care may not always be those that look the tidiest on paper.

Visionary leadership can therefore be linked with strategic management because, as well as pursuing operational management that gets the job done, an organisation needs an overall strategy or direction. Westley and Mintzberg (1991) suggest that visionary leadership is far more than a process of having an idea, conveying it to staff and seeing that it is carried through.

First, they see the whole process as needing to be *dynamic* and *interactive,* not purely top-down. We saw in Chapter 3 how important involvement and two-way communication are to motivating staff. In visionary management, the emphasis is on language that fires people up, on an active rather than a passive audience who are ready to be engaged and to take the new ideas into their day-to-day work, on repeating the message in different ways and helping people to take it on board, and on building mutual trust and empowerment through shared enthusiasm. Westley and Mintzberg use the analogy of a theatrical performance that sweeps its audience up into the drama. All good managers, like good teachers, have something of the performer about them and they certainly need charisma, although they also need integrity – a genuine belief in what they are saying. Interestingly to social workers, the theatrical metaphor makes it clear that there is a strong emotional content as well as a task focus in the conveying of a leadership message to an organisation. And the organisation has to be 'in the mood' to hear it; where staff feel undervalued, badly treated and disgruntled, they are unlikely to be swept up into anything except discontent and opposition to change.

Second, both *content* and *context* are important: the leader must have the right idea at the right time or no one will listen. Third, as with everything we have looked at in this book, there must be *flexibility* in visionary style. Some ideas start with instant inspiration, others are carefully evolved according to the changing needs of the organisation. Either way, an intense and durable vision will find its way through committee procedures, project development groups, translation into operational functioning on the ground and other organisational paraphernalia so as to make a difference to the way the organisation works and the service it gives to the public.

A strategy becomes more, then, than the single first idea. Mintzberg (see Moore, 1992) has shown that, whether the strategy emerges inspirationally or is deliberated upon in an incremental way, it has to be translated into a *plan* – a consciously intended course of action – and a pattern of *consistent behaviours* that carry through the plan. In a sense, a strategy is an abstraction but it becomes real when it is translated into action. So, just as every organisation needs a vision (a sense of where it is aiming to get to), so every vision needs a strategy that sets out the behaviours and actions needed to realise it. The strategy must be supported by an operational plan or nothing will actually happen. This plan specifies how the strategy will be implemented, in terms of human, financial and information resources, individual responsibilities and a timescale. And every plan requires *monitoring* and *evaluation* to find out whether it is being implemented and whether it is having the desired effect.

Strategy

For our purposes, *strategy* refers to the long-term actions and behaviours that are intended to make a reality of the vision for the organisation, setting out specific objectives and intended outcomes, in the form of measurable targets, and specifying the financial, human and other resources that will be needed. Drucker's (1954) listing of the seven tasks of the manager of tomorrow starts from managing by objectives and adds: taking risks further ahead and lower down the organisation; making strategic decisions; building an integrated and self-monitoring team; communicating rapidly and clearly to motivate others and engage their participation; taking an organisational overview including his or her own part in it; and informing decisions and actions from an international and sociopolitical perspective.

Strategic planning at its most basic is simply about setting *organisational objectives* and then *mobilising available resources* and the *integrated activity of staff* to achieve those objectives. In social welfare, this means shaping services in the light of law and policy, and managing the practice that delivers the policy. Strategy can be broken down into steps (McKenna and Beech, 1995):

- defining *corporate philosophy and mission statement,* setting out the overall values of the organisation and what purpose it exists to serve
- systematically analysing the *current social context* and the *political and economic climate* in which the organisation's welfare services are currently being delivered (including demographic trends, changes in welfare policy and advances in communication technology, the 'going rate' for costs and charges nationally, the current best practice in making services more acceptable and accessible to minority groups of services users)
- evaluating any *advantages* or *limitations* that the organisation itself may have.

These last two steps add up to a SWOT analysis, with the organisational strengths and weaknesses being set against environmental threats and opportunities (see Figure 4.1).

On the basis of all this information and clear thinking about overall purpose, the next steps are:

- developing *objectives and goals* for the organisation that will fulfil its mission

Figure 4.1 SWOT analysis

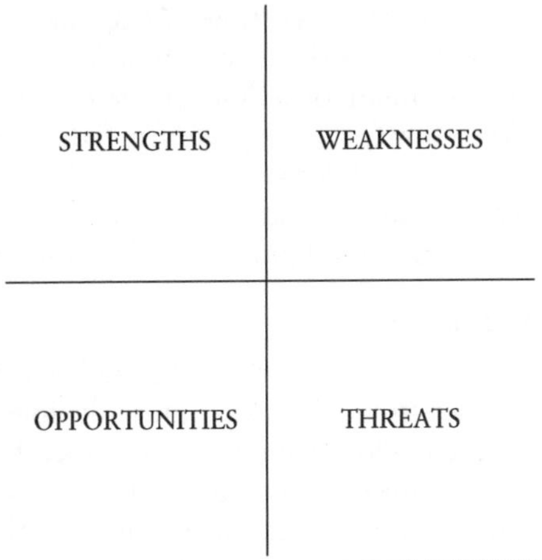

--------------		-------------
STRENGTHS		WEAKNESSES
OPPORTUNITIES		THREATS

- developing *detailed strategies designed to meet the targets over time,* sometimes jointly with other organisations, including through any planned change of direction, changes in operating systems or processes, or human resource policies
- building in *contingency plans* to cope with any unforeseen events or emergencies
- thinking about the *overall profile and long-term effectiveness* of the organisation
- *implementing* the strategy and constantly *evaluating* it against the stated aims and targets.

The public and private sectors have both tended to place increasing reliance on effective top managers, viewing them as the key human resource and rewarding and developing them as the central factor in organisational success. While it is clear that a lack of leadership can seriously damage an organisation, we have seen that the extent to which this is due to the individual or the context is often far from clear. In service organisations, the quality and commitment of staff are equally important. Consequently, in Chapter 5 we discuss how vital staff selection and support can be. Certainly, in social work, the skills and knowledge of all frontline employees are vital.

It is also important to remember that setting out a series of strategic steps makes organisational management sound more orderly than it can ever be in practice, where ideas and responses to situations tend to emerge over time. Also, there are plenty of critiques of simplistic claims that decision-making is a rational and strategic process. A useful overview of these demonstrates that change is far from always eagerly confronted, it often happens incrementally, if at all, and decisions may well be compromised in the face of organisational constraints or top-level tendencies to resort to little more than 'muddling through' (Hill, 1997).

From strategy to structure

Organisational structures can range from highly complex, multi-layered beauracracies to much looser, more flexible arrangements (in the voluntary sector, for example). Over time, the looser structures can lose their innovative edge or organisational clarity. They may need reorganising around the edges, for example to regularise the way various projects relate to purchasing organisations, while also maximising autonomy in developing new forms of service that are responsive to the expressed needs of users. Overall, though, Handy (1995) considers that the pace and unpredictability of change will need managers who can think unconventionally and organisational forms in which they have freedom of movement.

The current trend in local government is towards 'joined-up services', with one corporate grouping drawing all key policy-making back into the centre. This might lend itself to some newer organisational forms in the future, better able to adjust to the identification of wholly new ways of meeting need, and the falling from favour of old-style ones. Handy identified, for example, a 'triple I' organisation based on *information, intelligence* and *ideas,* with executives, professionals and specialists all committed to constant learning and working in more egalitarian design or project teams, not as managers and subordinates. This feels a long way removed from the new managerialism in social services but, again, there are voluntary bodies that work more along these lines, for example those that come together to develop new services or to advise on allocating new forms of funding.

In social work, we need clear strategy and structure but we also have to look beyond them. As we saw in Chapter 3, top-down management has serious limitations. In the 'caring services', people are everything. The need to listen to staff and make them feel valued and involved – indeed, to regard them as the organisation's greatest asset – will only be recognised if responses to change and the means adopted to meet the objective of delivering high quality services also have well developed, bottom-up components. This involves remembering that staff are individual people, not depersonalised 'posts', that they have a variety of skills and strengths and that they need motivating in different ways to give of their best. As we shall see in Chapter 6, however, no one feels motivated unless there is a supportive environment which is free of harassment and bullying and is committed to tackling racism and sexism, as well as meeting staff care and development needs.

Operational planning

Logically, operational plans should be based on strategic ones; they should be short-range – about a year – and spell out specific goals. Aims and objectives should be positive, motivating and written in terms that members of staff can identify with and apply directly to their own work. They should also give a sense of constant improvement through being prioritised and should include a progression from the more immediately achievable to those which, although realistic, will require effort. There should be measurable outcomes set against defined timescales.

Operational planning now forces us to focus on key resource issues, as well as on levels of demand for each service, its quality standards and the consideration of alternative ways of providing care. For instance, home care organisers might be asked to check current and short-term plans by asking questions related to specific topics, as shown below:

1. *Care management*: What are your guidelines for undertaking needs assessment, that is, what do you assess and how is this done? When do you review user needs? What are your plans for constructing, monitoring and reviewing care packages?
2. *Organising your section*: Are you integrated with others in the department? Have you decided on the sizes of workload for your home care managers? Have you delegated sufficient authority to ensure flexible use of your workforce?
3. *Resources*: Do you have a financial plan which includes the development of the service over the next year? Have you

decided how you will allocate resources across your catchment area and communicated this to your budget holders?

Checklists like this demonstrate that operational planning is concerned with continuous monitoring and evaluation of service provision. It is obvious, too, that it is based on costing.

Because planning activity and managing finance are so inextricably linked, a brief outline of how budgets are formed and controlled follows. In fact, although there has been much talk of 'devolved budgets', it is still generally the case that senior managers agree and monitor resource allocation and expenditure. There has not been the devolving downwards of financial responsibility that some had advocated. Nevertheless, spending does have to be checked and accountability for it demonstrated by frontline staff and first line managers in a way that previous generations of social workers simply would not have recognised.

Financial planning

The process of drawing up a budget starts by examining the cost of maintaining existing provision and meeting new demands, whether these result from demographic changes (for example increasing numbers of older citizens) or new initiatives planned in previous years (for example a new day centre which opens in the financial year under review). Managers have to contain spending within overall financial targets, which, in turn, are balanced against all the other commitments of the organisation. Allocations for each service are subdivided under various 'heads'; thus the cost of residential care, for example, has heads for everything from staff wages to postage costs. Within this, some costs will be 'fixed' and inescapable, others will be 'variable' because volumes of service can be decided according to what can be afforded. 'Marginal' costs relate to one-off and special activities which are less relevant when planning the core budget.

The traditional form of financial planning is known as the *incremental approach*, so called because it builds up, year on year, by considering the difference between the current and the proposed budget. Another name for it is *historic budgeting* because it uses what has been spent in the past as the basis for what will be allocated in the future. With this model, the annual submission of a budget to a governing body uses the current year's budget as the building block on which the analysis of the next year's needs is based. Each line item can be accepted or reduced by chief officers or members of the committee who decide the overall resources likely to be available. Senior managers seeking adequate levels of resources to commission the services they need may tend to submit estimates beyond what they require if they know that in recent years amounts have been routinely cut. This can lead to complex second-guessing. Healthier organisations operate on a more open basis and it can be a sign that an organisation is potentially at risk when annual financial planning is preoccupied with game-playing of this kind.

When expenditure is running ahead of target, managers may decide either to reduce the services provided or to transfer resources from an underspent area. This process is known as *virement*. To some extent, managers may be allowed to do this without going back to consult the committee that fixed the budget, providing the sums involved are not large, the virement is broadly within the same area of service and monies are not transferred from the resources allocated for staffing costs, since the only common exception to the ability to move money between heads is the staffing budget. In most organisations, managers cannot transfer money into this without formal approval, largely because of the risks of entering into contractual commitments without proper scrutiny.

More and more, the new role of a social worker or care manager as answerable for expenditure demands a knowledge of accounting and operational planning. It certainly involves understanding both resource obligations and resource constraints and being able to appreciate, argue and, where possible, reconcile a range of divergent views, while balancing financial control against operational flexibility (Pettinger, 1997). Also, frontline managers may find themselves in the role of decision-makers in the allocation of funds to commission individual services. Alternatively, they themselves may be working for an organisation whose survival depends on obtaining funds from the local authority and other bodies through contracts or grants. There are specific skills involved in writing tenders for contracts and applications for grants, which include being able to itemise a budget, outline service standards and highlight the benefits that the commissioner of the service would obtain by engaging this particular contractor.

In summary, the provision of good services needs the most effective use of resources. This requires the integration of the management of activity and of finance. Managing budgets that involve purchasing services from several suppliers demands a thorough understanding of the market environment and trends in demand for services. This, in turn, requires a detailed knowledge of the make-up of the local community and likely changes in social needs. In its last year of operation, the Joint Review Team produced a web-based guide to financial management in social services that is still available (http://www.joint-reviews.gov.uk/money).

Leadership role and style

What make a 'good leader'? If people are asked to list the qualities of the best and worst leaders they have known, they produce a list something like that given below. An effective leader:

● is considerate, friendly, supportive, fair and objective
● is enthusiastic, builds confidence and inspires others
● gives credit where it is due, and appreciates suggestions and ideas
● encourages participation in decision-making
● lets the staff know what is expected of them
● sets specific goals, measures progress and gives concrete feedback
● is aware of training and development needs, across the whole team or organisation
● keeps everyone informed about decisions and developments
● acts decisively in sorting out work-related problems
● delegates authority and responsibility appropriately
● emphasises the importance of each person working at his or her best
● devises plans in advance, including for contingencies
● makes sure that the team coordinates its activities
● enables the team to get on with its work
● establishes contacts with outsiders to promote liaison
● represents the team's needs to senior managers and is persuasive in negotiations with them for resources, staffing allocations and so on
● helps to settle conflicts and disagreements among the team members

- takes action if people do not pull their weight or if they violate the rules
- does all the above for the administrative as much as the professional staff
- ensures the team occasionally has some fun together, as part of wider team-building.

The items in this list clearly combine personal qualities with organisational knowledge, participative values, and task and process skills (note the conjunction of knowledge, values and skills, as in all good social work). The recurring aspects of a good leader, in any work setting, include particularly well developed 'people skills', problem-solving abilities, and the capacity to think systemically within accepted organisational structures and channels.

Mintzberg (1973) has described the work of managers in relation to 10 roles, of which 'leader' is only one. He lists: three interpersonal roles – figurehead, leader, and liaison person with the outside world; three roles in gathering and passing on information internally and externally, which he calls monitor, disseminator and spokesperson; and four roles relating to decision-making, those of entrepreneur, disturbance handler (again internal or external, dealing with conflict or unexpected change), resource allocator and negotiator. The effective manager will combine all these roles into an integrated whole, resolving any 'role ambiguity' or 'role conflict' and emerging with 'role confidence', whereby the individual takes pride in the role held and feels his or her self-worth to be confirmed by it (Pettinger, 1997).

Theories of leadership effectiveness also attempt to engage with the best style to adopt under particular circumstances, adapting it to deal effectively with the *task* (the job to be done) as well as the *people* dimensions (satisfying the needs of team members and the individuals within the team), bearing in mind the *situation* which faces us. And, these days, we want to keep the 'customer', or service user, to the fore. As we have already seen with organisational structures and management principles, it is impossible to dictate what works best overall or give one magic set of answers. So much nowadays is down to flexibility.

Leadership variables include *trait* (any personal qualities we may have, such as persistence), *style* (for example person-oriented or task-oriented, laissez-faire, authoritarian or democratic) and *situation* (the set of circumstances facing the leader or manager at the time). Leadership style can be conceptualised according to characteristics, such as the degree of emphasis on each of the following:

● compliance with rules and procedures, although, increasingly, there is an expectation that these will be internalised, that is, the manager will believe in them, not just carry them out
● delegation of responsibility to others
● standards set and monitored in all aspects of the work
● rewards for excellence rather than criticism and blaming, or rewarding on grounds of seniority, favouritism or cronyism
● distance maintained through managerial aloofness or reduced over time by building warm and trusting relationships with team members.

Managers can work out their own managerial style by asking themselves whether, in accordance with the above list, they have arrived at a point where:

● procedures are sufficiently well organised that people can be left to get on with their jobs but not so constraining as to hinder initiative
● staff are encouraged to take responsibility and 'own' their own decisions and initiatives without too much risk of mistakes, with manageable and comfortable limits on delegated power
● standards are not set too high or too low (or neglected altogether)
● everyone is regularly praised, and rewarded and criticised fairly
● there is a friendly and comfortable working atmosphere in which people can ask for support or advice when they need it.

Clearly, these aspects of style interact. In a high risk job like social work, people are not comfortable if there is too little monitoring of standards or too few checks and balances on procedures, but they also resent being treated like technicians rather than professionals. Above all, the manager has to try and understand how each team member (for a senior manager, this will be the management team) perceives their level of involvement with the organisation and the work in hand. The ideal is to maintain a balanced focus on both task and people aspects of the work (see Chapter 7 for more comment on 'masculine' and 'feminine' styles of communicating and working with others), with the ability to move along the autocratic–democratic

Figure 4.2 Continuum of leadership behaviour

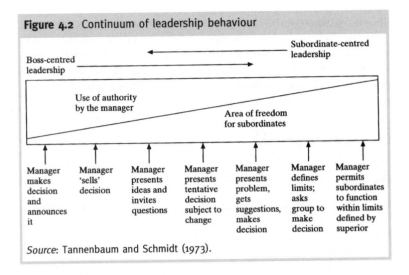

Source: Tannenbaum and Schmidt (1973).

axis as occasion demands. To exemplify this idea, Figure 4.2 shows a spectrum of seven behaviours or leadership styles. Moving from left to right, the area of freedom for the team increases.

Leadership, then, is not just a question of a fixed personal style. With practice, it should emerge from the balance of role, style, task, relationship with the team and the situation being faced (Payne, 2000). A well established leader, trusted by the group, will be able to adopt a democratic stance, encouraging people to be highly participative, and well placed to delegate with confidence. On the other hand, a new leader, or one with a poor relationship with the team and no real influence, will be in a difficult position, particularly if the task is unclear or highly complex. In such circumstances, it is often wise to focus on the job, not the relationship with the team, even if a democratic style is normally preferred. The situation may require telling people what to do for a time, while trying to persuade and motivate the team towards goal achievement. As with so much in management, flexibility is the key.

Hersey and Blanchard (1982) have further pointed out that another situational variable is the *maturity of the team*. The concept of 'maturity' is a nebulous one, but a group's psychological maturity might be portrayed, for instance, by their willingness to help one another. (In groupwork with service users, we recognise the strengths of a developed group as one where there is strong commitment, open relationships and balanced perspectives.) On top of this is *task maturity* (that is, being able to do the job). Working with a defensive team, for example, a person-centred style may not work and the manager who has only one leadership style to call upon will be in trouble.

Using power responsibly

A common classification into seven bases of power was set out by French and Raven (1959) and modified by later writers:

● *reward power*: the ability of the leader to give and take away praise, funding, promotion, resources and so on
● *coercive power*: the ability to reprimand and discipline, also to withhold career development opportunities
● *legitimate power*: conferred by position or office held in the organisation; a Weberian idea – see Chapter 2
● *expert power*: the use of superior skills and knowledge
● *referent power*: this is closely tied to charisma, where others desire to seek the leader's approval.

To this list are added *information* or *gatekeeper power*, where we become interested in having the information others keep to themselves, and *connection power* – having contact with influential people within the organisation.

As well as asking themselves which of these kinds of power they now possess (and what kinds the others in the hierarchy are using), new managers also have to question the degree of *perceived power* they hold and whether others are vying for it. Informal leaders, for example, act as if they are powerful even though they do not have the organisational authority to back them up, while some actual, appointed leaders allow others to usurp their influence by defaulting on the exercise of their authority and responsibilities. Furthermore, power does not only operate top-down. Everyone in the team has access to negative power, for example, which can be operated through such means as deliberate absenteeism, delaying urgent work or stalling in the implementation of improved practices. The effective manager may well have to tackle some of these phenomena, perhaps as part of changing the overall culture of the workplace.

Power can, then, be both used and abused. If managers are to harness their position in order to become effective leaders, it is vital that they do not exploit their authority and are particularly aware of the ethical aspects of decision-making. The responsible use of power cannot be taken as given merely because people are working in the human and public services. Codes of ethics and good conduct are as quickly forgotten in management as they can be in direct service provision. As social workers, we are still capable of being less than humane in our approach to each other and service users. There are also deviant ways of acquiring power and exercising it. Some people may gravitate to senior positions in order to fulfil a need to control others; they are more likely to be overbearing and bullying in manner, and to manage by fear rather than by mutual respect. Equally, others do not feel comfortable holding power and may attempt to minimise what it means, perhaps leaving all decisions to the team and counting on group norms to maintain standards. These are stereotypically 'masculine' and 'feminine' styles, although both men and women can be observed operating in either style (see Chapter 7).

For the manager who wants to make a show of his or her power, the contemporary fascination with surface appearance opens up all the possibilities of power dressing, wielding the mobile phone and so on. But there are more subtle ways of winning respect. For those who are underselling themselves in the power stakes, it may feel more acceptable to think about increasing influence rather than increasing power. With subordinates, it is possible to encourage others to do what you want by creating certain norms and carrying these through with personal authority (thus using 'normative', rather than 'coercive' or 'remunerative' power). With those higher in the hierarchy, personal presentation is still an issue but it has to mean creating a style that is personally comfortable, not necessarily wearing dark suits or teetering on ever higher heels. It also involves correcting negative verbal and non-verbal signals, such as not apologising when beginning to speak, not fiddling nervously, and making eye contact more often. Some of the more job-oriented ideas for increasing personal influence within the organisation include:

- consciously taking on key roles or projects
- saying 'no' to things that will have no personal pay-off and should be done by more junior people

- joining and fostering influential networks
- making presentations at high-profile meetings
- taking office in key groups
- documenting achievements
- developing skills that other people need to call upon
- taking advantage of presentational and personal effectiveness courses
- assisting the team to perform to a high standard and win accolades
- doing favours for people in order to be able to call on them in turn when in need of help
- being flexible, which means only ever standing on one's dignity or holding to a fixed stance if one's position would otherwise become untenable.

These are all ways of becoming more visible and hence more influential without overstating one's claims or being underhand. In these days of multi-agency partnerships, it can also be a good idea to be the person who undertakes key aspects of liaison, although not by becoming so specialised as to become marginalised and dispensable (Balloch and Taylor, 2001). None of these suggestions is restricted to SSDs or even to paid posts. The trustee or volunteer committee member of a charity, for example, may be equally interested in developing a power base from which to influence the future direction of the organisation's work.

In order to have time to think in this broader way and take on the additional tasks involved, it is vital to be able to *delegate*. Otherwise a manager is likely to become bogged down in the day-to-day work of the team in inappropriate ways. The essentials of delegation include:

- creating a culture of participation and mutual respect
- using staff development opportunities to maximise the abilities of all team members
- trusting staff to exercise those abilities
- building this gradually into career opportunities for people so that they will welcome the new experience and extra work
- providing considerable support when people take on a new task and reducing this to some extent over time
- building in checks and balances so that people cannot run on too far without errors or poor decisions becoming visible, for

example regular reports to the manager, careful monitoring of all forms of management information by other relevant people
- allowing people to learn from misjudgements without suffering unreasonable penalties – or they will never try again
- never doing other people's work for them.

The one exception to the last 'rule' is where someone is in immediate danger or an unsafe working practice requires instant rectification. Burton (1998) gives the example of mopping the dangerously slippery floor in the residential home lavatory oneself, assuming that the person who normally does it is not immediately to hand and free to do it, *before* putting one's manager's hat back on and going to find out how it came to be left like that and how this can be avoided in future. (An 'out of order' sign might do instead!)

Overall, it should be the end product and the performance standard that matter, not (within limits) how the staff member achieves these; they may well have a very different working method and should be given the freedom to pursue it. Structuring in progress reports will provide reassurance along the way. Delegation can fruitfully build on the staff's own interests but should also challenge people to learn new knowledge and skills, otherwise people will not develop in the rounded way that will equip them to seek advancement in due course. (It is noticeable, for example, that people tend to ask to go on courses about things they already know about and can do well, that is, in their areas of special interest, not their areas of weakness where new learning might help most.) In delegating, we are, after all, also mentoring and coaching more junior employees. Finally, the more people who can see a task through as a self-contained project, and understand its relevance to the organisation's work as a whole, and the more they can draw on information and guidance from the sources the manager him- or herself would have used, the more they will feel empowered to do a good job and the more the whole team will benefit.

Although there will always be business conducted and discussions held in the gents' loo or the changing room (where not all of us can go), and although subcultures and cliques to which we do not all belong and unspoken rules and expectations we are not all party to will persist, it should still be possible to be noticed doing a good job and be rewarded for it. Perhaps it is akin to presenting oneself at work like a walking CV, not afraid to say what you have done and what you are good at. And it is often to the benefit of the team and the organisation when a manager does well; remembering this may make it easier to adopt a less self-effacing style.

Some of the situations in which people do acquire too much power or abuse it are where:

- there are loose supervision arrangements and few external controls
- an organisation is undergoing change (decentralising its operations, for instance) and is temporarily destabilised
- control is gained over critical resources, be it by one manager having sole say over allocating resources, or an administrator holding the key to the stationery cupboard
- the employee is an expert in a needed field and does not share this knowledge, for example the mystery surrounding computer know-how
- obligations are created so that others feel beholden.

The manager who observes an abuse of power by another may find it easier to start by considering how to alter the situation in which the power has been assumed or has apparently become legitimised, for example by analysing it according to the above list, rather than by personally confronting the individual concerned as the first course of action taken. The ideas in Chapter 3 on managing change might also be useful, for example in seeking allies who have noticed the same problem and who would cooperate to solve it, or in considering what aspects of the current situation are maintaining the status quo and which could be used to change it (as in a force field analysis). Where there is harassment of staff or an unacceptable response to service users, however, the more formal channels to take action against the person concerned may have to be used straight away. It may be helpful to think about this in terms of 'standard', 'discretionary' and 'forbidden' areas of power. There is a difference between those people who are doing a job we do not happen to like, those who are exercising their room for manoeuvre in slightly unpleasant ways and those who are actually perpetrating some form of misconduct. It may also be possible to seek confidential advice from a human resources manager without naming the person who is causing concern, before deciding what to do. As soon as dissatisfaction is voiced about someone or action taken against them, some options begin to close down and others open up, so it is as well to have thought things through in advance.

The use of *persuasion* deserves a final word as a potent (if overlooked) skill when used responsibly. Persuasion relies on: being able to communicate effectively; knowing how to monitor and control one's own tone and behaviour; monitoring and thus maximising other people's understanding and acceptance, including by finding out what matters most to them; and consciously conveying a relaxed, calm manner. It is often possible to influence others, including in multidisciplinary settings, by offering a single, firm proposal (we have to know what we want before we can get others to want it); building on this, and coping with disagreements like 'It won't work' in an open way; welcoming the voicing of concerns by other people and talking them through fully, not blocking their expression; testing for understanding; giving and seeking information; and summarising the points being made by all parties. Again, we saw many of these ideas in Chapter 3, in relation to managing change.

Leadership and management tasks

Control

The task we tend to think of as synonymous with management is that of controlling the work of others on behalf of the wider organisation. To the newly appointed, first-time manager, this will be an unfamiliar responsibility, sometimes more difficult than just getting on and doing the work oneself. But, of course, the latter is no longer possible because there is not time to do both. The number of staff who report directly to the manager is called the 'span of control' (see Chapter 2). The more rigid the hierarchy, the smaller the span, but 'leaner, fitter' organisations have been shedding middle-tier managers, thus making spans wider. In social work, managers do not have the freedom to appoint their own deputies to help them with their workload, but they can feed into reviews of staffing structures where there is clearly too much work to do and also seek to have staff seconded or allocated to carry out particular projects where important tasks would otherwise not get done.

Of course, the manager should not be left to tell others what to do on a whim. All manner of mechanisms and requirements will have been established by the organisation to ensure that people are operating within the agreed policies and their work is overseen effectively. This increasingly happens within a performance management framework. As a new manager, it is well worth getting hold of all available written procedures, policies and other documentation, as well as identifying the key administrators within the organisation who are responsible for their oversight and can advise on when and how to apply them in practice. The normal internal monitoring channels will include financial forecasts, reports and audits, management information on service delivery and staffing matters, feeding into committee reports on specific topics, feedback to one's peers and one's own managers, conflict resolution mechanisms (see below) and periodic overviews of particular areas of work (Pettinger, 1997).

There are also external procedures to which all managers are answerable. For local authorities, these have included Joint Reviews by the SSI and the Audit Commission (Jones, 1999c) and will in future encompass inspections by the National Commission for Care Standards (NCCS) and equivalents in the rest of the UK. An integrated approach to the inspection of children's services will be adopted by the Audit Commission, the NCCS and others, led by Ofsted. Consultation with local service users and carers constitutes a growing part of all such exercises, with service users (including young people) involved as inspectors. Service users are also well represented on the governing bodies of the new regulatory councils, as well as more fully consulted by local authorities as a key element of establishing 'Best Value'. It is probable that external inspection of major service areas will increasingly be undertaken by teams from two or more inspectorates, reflecting a partnership approach and based on a focus on the experience of the service user and not the operation of the organisation as an end in itself.

A new form of regulation of staff was implemented in the UK in 2002 with the creation of the General Social Care Council (GSCC) in England and the respective Social Care/Services Councils in Scotland, Wales and Northern Ireland. These bodies are responsible for: approving the qualifications of social workers; maintaining a register of qualified social workers and social care staff; dealing with complaints against individual registered practitioners, including through disciplinary proceedings; enforcing sanctions against registered practitioners who have broken the code of conduct (including the possibility of removing a person from the register, which would remove their opportunity to work in the field); and also promoting social care and social work. The GSCC has published a Code of Practice for individual practitioners and employers (http://www.gscc.org.uk/codes_practice.htm), which forms the basis of these procedures.

Within an overall project to 'modernise' social services (DoH, 1998a), regulations and standards are increasingly being set nationally by central government. The ultimate sanction for serious or persistent failure to meet them, under the Local Government Act 1999, is government intervention to hand responsibility for running the department to, for example, a neighbouring local authority. This inevitably creates additional pressures on managers in expecting all staff to meet externally determined requirements and monitoring the extent to which this is achieved. It also means that managers nowadays are less often involved in setting standards from scratch, except in relation to particular quality or change management initiatives (see Chapter 3), and more often in measuring continuous improvement against externally determined criteria.

In the field of child care, for example, the government's Quality Protects initiative (DoH, 1998b) is based on published national objectives that local authorities are required to meet, together with more detailed sub-objectives and exhaustive performance indicators to measure outcomes for children. These tend to be numerical in nature, aiming, for example, to increase by half the number of children in care leaving school with at least one GCSE pass and minimise the waiting time in care before adoption (DoH, 1999).

While no one would question the government's aim of improving children's life chances, it is questionable whether such a mechanistic and regulated approach can truly respond to the qualitative aspects of their lives. For example, a rush to get children adopted can lead to separating sibling groups and eroding contact arrangements (Mullender, 1999). The numerical measures themselves are also open to criticism; why, for instance, should children only be expected to gain one GCSE pass just because they cannot live with their own families (*Community Care*, 14–20 October 1999)? Similarly, the checklists in the LAC documentation may impose middle-class norms instead of capturing the diversity of family and community expectations and of young people's own identities (Garrett, 1999). Standards in other fields, such as the government's performance indicators for adult services and national service framework for mental health, are open to equivalent criticism, while the whole idea of setting standards as a way of improving working relationships between social services and the voluntary sector, in the form of a 'compact', is perhaps a little strained (Thompson, 1999). Nevertheless, such a compact now exists and has its own benchmarks, which require the statutory sector, among other things, to build in voluntary sector participation in planning and delivering services, make proper internal organisational arrangements to ensure that this happens, and review and evaluate the results.

The expectations introduced across the whole of social services work in local authorities, in the form of a Performance Assessment Framework (DoH, 1999), cover strategic objectives, costs and efficiency, effectiveness of service delivery, quality of services and access to them for both children and adults. Inevitably, all such attempts to regularise and standardise practice through national priorities and objectives create more administration and bureaucracy at the local level. For the manager, an emphasis on outcomes imposes fresh pressures and additional work because the changes are being introduced within a management-led model and, not least, because 'league tables' are now published as to how local authorities perform. However, this does at least offer clarity as to precisely what is demanded, where previously there may have been only a vague sense of 'must try harder' or of the goalposts shifting with every external inspection or audit. It does also generally bring an influx of resources, for example the special grant for children's services that was payable for three years until 2001–2, and, even if this was largely intended to pay for the information-gathering and outcome measurement involved, these are vital to the organisation in tracking what is actually happening to children in the LAC system. It is also an important advance that the social care workforce is now being regulated for the first time, with recognition of qualifications, codes of conduct for all staff and removal or suspension from the register of those considered unsafe to practise (Jones, 1999b). The imposition of central directives upon standards is therefore probably best described as a mixed blessing.

Conflict resolution and dealing with disciplinary matters

It has been estimated that managers in business and industry spend up to 20 per cent of their time resolving conflict (Anderson, 1985).

They are not alone. Staff in group care, for example, who work in close proximity with one another and often with service users' distress, may encounter a considerable amount of it, too. Early theorists such as Weber and Taylor, whose ideas were examined in Chapter 2, viewed conflict as undesirable and believed that it destroyed morale. More recent thinking suggests that this depends on the amount of conflict and how it is managed (Fisher and Ury, 1983). Disagreements might assist problem-solving and hence should be dealt with rather than suppressed. Challenges can be creative if well managed.

The organisation as a whole will have procedures and regulations to ensure equity and clarity for staff and service users, communication channels to air issues that need resolving, and managers in fields such as human resources who can advise on rights, precedents and problem-solving tactics. The agency will also have mechanisms in place for dealing with serious eventualities such as harassment, grievances and disciplinary matters. The line manager's role is to try and ensure that problems are dealt with without needing to go through any of these channels – and not simply by keeping the lid on any area of difficulty. Indeed, a manager can usefully spot trouble brewing by noticing that someone's performance is declining or that morale is low in the team. Higher than average staff turnover or sickness absence can also be indicators that all is not well.

The manager's first task on suspecting a problem is to identify where the disagreement or dissatisfaction is occurring and why. In almost all cases, staffing difficulties, just like complaints from service users, are best handled as near to the problem as possible, by the first line manager.

The dual aims of a manager are to resolve the conflict if at all possible, while maintaining a working relationship with the people concerned. If a manager responds to conflict by ignoring it or withdrawing, she or he loses on both counts since avenues of communication are shut off as people build up resentments. Alternatively, someone who forces a resolution can thereby lose their working relationship with those who are obliged to comply. Smoothing or suppressing conflict could maintain the relationship but does not fulfil the other aim of resolving the problem. A compromise or bargaining approach accomplishes the two aims but, later, the parties to the conflict may feel that they gave in too much. Thus, securing an outcome which resolves the conflict and keeps relationships intact requires positively confronting and being honest with people. To reach this optimal position, management texts exhort us to see conflict as an *opportunity* rather than a problem – frustrations have to be reframed as chances to 'clear the air'. Although we saw in Chapter 2 that this thinking has been around for a century or so, it may be easier said than done, especially for those of us brought up to be overly polite or to fear retaliation. Additionally, getting involved can be draining of one's energies for other tasks. But it *is* true that conflict signals the impetus for change, as we know from groupwork and crisis intervention with service users as well as from management experience.

When the opposing parties are brought together, the skills are, first, to reveal the issues. This is done by: deciding what the conflict is really about; distinguishing between people's values, wants and needs; working at getting people to understand one another's way of looking at things and to overcome their own anger in order to become empathic; and exposing discrepancies in definitions of the problem. Conflicts may arise from matters as wide ranging as the organisation, the way work is organised within it, industrial relations, management style, or an individual's own values or beliefs (Pettinger, 1997). It may be ideological, career-related or job-related. Any conflict involves clarifying who are the parties to the conflict, what is actually at issue, the dynamics of the situation (including what has happened up to this point and what it will take to put it right), and the best way for management to respond in order either to remove the causes of the conflict, or to contain and control it so that it does not cause damage, or to harness it into some useful energy for change. Uncontrolled conflict is often a sign of poor management on a wider scale.

Having 'rolled out' the issues, the next tasks comprise:

- separating the people from the problem
- jointly teasing out multiple, creative options for problem-solving
- getting to the real source of the problem so as to eliminate it (for instance, great conflict ensued when residents in a home for people with learning difficulties were allowed to make their own drinks and sometimes had accidents; the issue was really a difference of staff opinion about dependence/independence goals)

- seeking a 'win–win' outcome in preference to one with winners and losers
- knowing that every situation is unique and judging, therefore, whether to use the strategy of ignoring the conflict, or of smoothing it over, or of actively confronting it.

More serious is the process for formal disciplinary action, which, although matters are handled by senior managers, almost invariably starts with a decision by the immediate manager. All managers therefore need to internalise the procedures, since any staff member at any time could become the subject of, or witness to, an enquiry. Disciplinary procedures are designed to encourage an unsatisfactory employee to improve, if they are failing or having difficulties in work, so as to safeguard the rights of service users and/or other staff. It is clearly necessary for social work agencies to have such systems in place in order to ensure that standards are maintained and service users are protected. The quasi-judicial nature of this duty may cause some managers sufficient unease for them to avoid taking action even when it is sorely needed. Or they may take inappropriate action such as continually sending the poor performer on courses or moving them around different teams, long after it is clear that this will not bring them up to standard, in the hope that someone else will take the decision to fail them and draw attention to their shortcomings. Social work is a 'caring profession' and has been caricatured as 'soft' or weak, especially when dealing with personnel problems. However, social workers have to take tough decisions about rights, liberty and behaviour in their daily work. We know that it is not a sign of caring to leave someone unassisted who cannot manage alone or to ignore unacceptable behaviour. The same applies in personnel matters. It is ultimately unethical to let a member of staff struggle on in a post to which they are unsuited and in which they are causing harm to others. If attempts to solve the problem with a staff development or staff care approach (see Chapter 6) have failed, then disciplinary measures may be needed. Useful information on these matters is available from ACAS, whose general approach is summarised below. Above all, it is important to work with the human resources manager.

Employees should be given the opportunity to involve their trade union and/or professional association at an early stage. This provides independent support for the individual but also helps the organisation to follow the formal procedure. A failure to follow procedures can prove costly, should an individual win an appeal against their employer for discrimination or failure to follow due process. An independent advocate can also help the individual to look at the reality of what has happened and to argue their case most effectively.

The first stage is always to ensure that the individual knows there is a problem and precisely what it is, and to obtain his or her own view and explanation. In order to observe the principles of natural justice, senior managers should:

- ensure that they could not be accused of bias or involvement, that is, that they are the right person to deal with the case
- gather all the relevant information promptly before memory fades
- take statements and collect documents and records of any previous warnings, together with evidence of their impact or lack of it and accurate dates wherever possible
- be clear about the complaint and make sure this form of action is necessary (in some cases the employee might be willing to accept internal or external help to overcome a problem within an agreed timescale, or may elect to resign)
- prepare carefully for any disciplinary interview and advise the person of their rights, giving time for the person initially to state and then to prepare to defend her/his case
- consider adjourning the hearing before reaching a decision on any penalty
- finally, inform the individual of the decision and the reasons for it, record the action and monitor its implementation.

Besides careful preparation for a disciplinary interview and making sure that an employee has time to prepare his or her case, managers need to arrange for a time and place where there will be no interruptions, and to ensure that someone takes notes and that, if required, an interpreter is available. It is important for the manager who is chairing the interview to start by explaining its purpose and how it will be conducted (even though it may not run to plan if feelings are running high) and to introduce everyone by name and role. Then he or she should state precisely what the complaint is about, obtain the employee's reply and any witnesses' comments, encourage general questioning and discussion (adjourning if necessary at any point), ensure that the employee has a full and fair hearing, and summarise the main points of the alleged shortcoming before adjourning to take a decision so as to allow proper consideration of all the matters raised. As chair, he or she should remain firm but polite throughout.

In the case of a minor misdemeanour, the individual should be given a formal oral warning and measures put in place to prevent a recurrence. Where the problem is more serious or there has been an accumulation of minor failings, a formal written warning should be given. Further misconduct or unsatisfactory performance may warrant a final written warning. Because there may be these various stages to go through, it is important to take action promptly and to record the salient details along the way. Suspension without pay and dismissal require further guidance, and, again, advice from the human resources manager regarding rights on the termination of employment should be sought. In the personal social services, in the case of gross misconduct such as abuse of a service user or dishonesty, an immediate final warning or dismissal may be appropriate in order to protect the public. An appeal can be made at each stage of the procedure.

It is not surprising, perhaps, that at times staff are relieved when action such as this is taken as a way of trying to improve the performance of, or occasionally remove, a difficult colleague. The aim, after all, is reformative, not punitive. One manager's team effusively thanked him for finally doing something. In another case, a skilled and talented employee decided not to leave her job when her harasser was formally confronted about his behaviour, at which time other problems with his work also began to emerge. Had no action been taken, the good worker would have gone and the problematic one would have remained, unchecked. More usually, though, the failing is a minor one and is unnoticed or 'carried' by the team, such as making too many private telephone calls, poor timekeeping, inaccurate word processing and so on. What do we do? Most managers dread having to tell someone off, while a few bullies get an inappropriate kick out of it.

The dynamics of oppression may make it more difficult to deal with these matters, not only in cases where the manager (being white and male, say) could be accused of oppressing the staff member (if black and/or female), but also where, for example, a black senior social worker or one who is considerably younger than the team member in question cannot assume that they will be respected or listened to. Being assertive is part of the skill of being an effective manager, rather than being passive/aggressive in relating to team members. But, here too, there is an interplay with oppression. At one assertiveness training workshop, for example, a black woman officer-in-charge said she had tried being assertive in her job but had been misperceived as aggressive and awkward. A female senior probation officer at the same event had found that all her team had seen her as 'bossy' when she quite properly instructed a team member to bring records up to date.

Above all, one has to make clear not only the behaviour that offends and why, but what is expected of the worker in terms of improvement and of the team as a whole in terms of acceptable standards of performance. Not only is this fair to the individual employee, but groups, including teams, perform better when they see everyone treated alike, with no favoured colleagues and no mood swings on the part of the team or group leader that mean a behaviour is acceptable one day and not the next.

Nowadays, it is not only managers who need these skills but all workers. Implementing care plans, for example, may involve monitoring contract compliance on the part of a service provider or overseeing the work of a volunteer. If confrontation is necessary, it helps to be aware of the other person's emotional state without letting one's own emotions run out of control. Time spent thinking what to say beforehand helps one to cope better. Second, dissatisfactions are best voiced at the time they are felt, otherwise they may become disconnected from the specific behaviours that offend and appear as a personal hobby horse. The focus should be on specific, unacceptable standards and conduct of work. Sticking to the problem, staying firm, and avoiding personalised attacks will help most staff to accept constructive criticism. Third, another important tip is always to be ready (once the initial problem has been stated) to explore what might help put things right. Again, most people can recognise reasonable suggestions as helpful, provided they are not in a state of anger or other heightened emotion at the time (which might make it preferable to return to the subject on another occasion). But it is important to build into this an agreed means of monitoring future performance, with a stated timescale and so on, so as not to be 'fobbed off' with promises of improvement which are not then carried through. Fourth, an offer to help solve the difficulty, emphasising the person's good points, is useful, as is a statement that one does not harbour grudges. It is important for a manager to be seen to be consistent and fair; unequal treatment, as we have said, is soon picked up by the team.

One tip that can prove helpful is to offer the other person a way out, and never, ever to back them into a corner where their only options are to respond with defensiveness or attack, rather than through logical problem-solving. This technique is useful because it leads to a 'win–win' situation where the desired end is obtained without anyone losing face. It can be particularly helpful when having to challenge someone more powerful than oneself within the organisation because it focuses on a possible solution rather than on an apparent challenge to their overall authority and presents them with a problem you have already half sorted out.

Finally on this subject, we do clearly recognise that there can also be grave abuses perpetrated in social care settings, such as physical and/or sexual abuse of service users, intimidation and the inappropriate use of power. Complaints procedures, appraisal mechanisms to oversee the work of staff and much clearer performance standards generally (including where service providers carry out work under contract) are all intended to help gather the evidence of unsatisfactory performance where necessary. It is also the case that whistleblowers will occasionally quite properly draw attention to serious problems that somehow have fallen through all these safety nets and they have certain legislative protection in doing so (Hunt, 1998). Part of the manager's role may then be to ensure that the person who 'blows the whistle' does not come off worse than the person who has been causing the problems because others close ranks around the accused party. Some of the problems that come to light may actually have taken place some years before, as in child abuse scandals in residential care, when there was less oversight of standards and more scope for individual exploitation of position (and, of course, less awareness of the prevalence of abuse). But abuses do continue to occur and managers continue to have to face the pressures of dealing with them, assisted, fortunately, by increasingly clear procedures.

Conducting meetings

Social workers often feel as if they spend their lives in meetings. If, after two or three hours, we are left wondering what we have achieved, we will find ourselves wishing they were chaired more thoughtfully. In a recent instance encountered by one of the authors, for example, the chair had not ensured that all the necessary people were in attendance (or contacted for information in advance) and almost every item had to be deferred. In this way, he wasted the time of everyone there.

Social workers go to many kinds of meetings, such as work allocation meetings, ward rounds or regular staff meetings. Occasionally, there are additional task group meetings set up for special projects. At one time, these acquired a particularly bad name, with workers saying of a problem that was inevitably going to be shelved: 'Let's set up a working party!' The advice offered below about more routine meetings could also avoid some of the wasted effort among ad hoc groups.

An effective chair of a meeting will do all the following:

1. Ensure that a meeting is really necessary and that the matters could not be resolved by a memo, a circular with a response deadline, telephone or email, or by seeing one or two key people separately.
2. Make sure that the size of the meeting is workable for the intended purpose; about 12 people is a maximum if everyone is to take part (otherwise, scan the agenda to see if everyone has to be present for each item).
3. Indicate on the agenda the function each item is intended to fulfil (for example, 'for information', 'for discussion', or 'for decision').
4. Make the agenda items self-explanatory, not vaguely stated as, say, 'Budget'.
5. Order the items in such a way that the meeting starts with a lively concern and, if possible, ends with one which unites the group.
6. State the starting and ending times.
7. Circulate the agenda and brief supporting papers, neither so far in advance that people lose them nor so late that they cannot read them in time for the meeting.
8. State at the outset what the meeting intends to achieve, assist in achieving these goals and keep his or her own intervention to a sentence or two on any item.
9. Always start the meeting on time.

10. Give prior thought to the order of agenda items. Meetings, however briskly chaired, are more likely to give full attention to items in roughly the middle two quarters of the agenda; they are not warmed up for the opening items and tend to rush through the last ones in order to get finished. The smart chair can select those issues that need the most consideration, as against others that need widespread agreement without protracted debate (for example where they have been 'done to death' in previous meetings).

11. Give clear signals that 'We must move on' or that it is someone else's turn to speak when any one person hogs the discussion.

12. Ensure that everyone understands the issues, writing on a board or flipchart (or asking someone else to do so) if the item involves details or needs analysing into separate parts.

13. Briefly summarise at the end of each item to help with minute-taking and show what has been achieved; also agree what action is to be taken, by whom and by when.

14. Perhaps bring senior people in to speak only after a wide spread of views is known so as to prevent the inhibition of junior staff.

15. End by agreeing the date, time and place of the next meeting in people's diaries to save contacting them later (or do this earlier in the meeting if anyone has to leave).

16. Regardless of who has been assigned to write the minutes, still take responsibility for ensuring that they are both accurate and complete before they are circulated, consulting the minute-taker about any changes.

17. Use the process of the meeting as well as its content to good effect, for example by helping the team to gel or to collaborate, giving a sense of collective identity, producing shared ideas and plans, showing where contributions mesh, improving commitment to the decisions and underlining the manager's role as (democratic) leader.

Finally, because we are always being prompted to be efficient, effective and able to justify expenditure, it is sometimes worth reckoning up how much meetings actually do cost in terms of travel and salary of those attending. So late arrivals, low participation and constantly deferred items have to be tackled. On the other hand, it can be a false saving of time not to have an item out fully while everyone is present. The trick is in recognising which issues require team discussion, fresh commitment, or change of direction so that they need to be brought to a meeting rather than circulated for information or individualised feedback. As electronic communication takes on more and more forms, it is also worth considering whether an agency-based or interagency meeting is absolutely necessary or whether a three-way phone call, a pre-arranged telephone conference, use of a mailbase on email, or even a video link-up could serve the same purpose.

Dealing with management information

Managing the day-to-day work of the team or organisation is only part of the story. Increasingly, it is recognised that an overview is needed over a period of time in order to plan ahead, meet targets, and improve on past performance where possible. This is where high quality management information comes in. Only the manager who is provided with up-to-date statistics and also 'softer' information on every relevant aspect of work and organisational infrastructure will be in a position to gauge how well staff are doing and where improvements are most urgently needed. Prioritising spending and effort relies on this background picture. When the topic of information is introduced, thoughts tend to turn immediately to computers and, certainly, producing the right statistical data, on time and in a usable format, is a key part of the process. But it is only one part. The existing software, or the uses to which it is put, may not be producing everything that the manager needs to know and, here, the manager's vision is essential in coming up with the right questions so that additional data can be produced – not all of it through crunching numbers, as we noted in Chapter 3. Working closely with the IT staff and other information systems managers to discuss what can be learned is important, as is making good appointments to such positions. There are many stories of interviewers being overly impressed with technical qualifications and jargon so that they have ended up employing people who are no good with people or who have no commitment to the overall work of the organisation.

In other words, information itself 'is a key resource which needs to be managed', as are those who produce and use it (NISW, 1996). Statistics are not necessarily reliable just because they are on paper in black and white, and all information can usefully be 'triangu-lated' with other sources of data, as is done in research. Standards of accuracy will vary according to how information is gathered (and by whom). It is only in relatively recent years, for example, that frontline staff have had to deal with financial assessments and financial targets or have had to input these details straight into the computer. This may well be a better system than maintaining mountainous case files that frequently lacked or obscured basic facts. But computers can get things wrong as well as people, espe-cially where a program has gone through many modifications. Here again, a good computer manager can advise.

It is also a good idea to work with internal and external auditors so as to learn what they require. They will have a good under-standing of what it is possible and reasonable to expect. At the wider level, authorities can club together to compare notes on base-line information to be able to set more realistic targets, charges and so on (*Community Care*, 14–20 January 1999, p. 6).

Overall, then, it is important to manage information rather than being managed by it (Sapey, 1997). This requires strategic and prin-cipled planning. At all levels, including basic grade practice, it is possible to move from seeing the data as a tool of management into regarding it as a helpful way of managing practice (NISW, 1996). This depends upon practitioners being given information outputs as well as being expected to make inputs. Staff themselves may come up with new ideas if they can see patterns of service take-up by different groups of users. They also always hold knowledge in their heads that is neither requested nor recorded by formal information channels. Sharing the management information picture with staff – the overall pattern of spending, the categories of users, priorities, needs and so on – and widening training beyond merely being able to input data into the computer can generate fruitful discussion at the team level, which may assist the organisation to rethink how effectively resources are dispensed and how user satisfaction rates can be increased.

A similar argument applies to sharing information with users and carers and with the wider public. Most people do not want to make unreasonable demands and want to be proud of the local services they help fund. Corporate newsletters telling residents what their council tax is spent on are commonplace but consulta-tion exercises that feed into planning services could all be far more of a two-way, information-sharing exercise. These questions of ownership have always been present in social work and the possession of good quality information could just as easily open them up as close them down. There is no intrinsic reason why managers should hide behind their sheets of numbers.

For the new manager, the starting point is not to be afraid of the information systems or the data they produce but to regard them as being there to serve the needs of managers, staff and service users. Precise and timely information about types and levels of need, the services available locally (in one's own organisation and beyond), costs, charges and financial targets, and staffing resources in one's own organisation are all invaluable. The manager has a right to discuss the format in which this material is presented and the use to which it is put, as well as a responsibility to educate the team about gathering and recording information accurately and about the potential, in turn, for using it to raise standards and sometimes for making working life easier. A good example of this can be using the data as a basis to argue for extra resources or changes of focus. It is still quite rare, for example, to record data on cases involving domestic violence and consequently even rarer to have designated staff in social services contexts to deal with the issue.

Decision-making

Decision-making is the process of choosing between possible courses of action and is therefore something we all do all the time. In management, it is of the essence, notably in relation to planning. Decisions may be arrived at unilaterally, by group or committee consensus, by a majority vote, through delegation, by a powerful minority or by default, that is, where there has been no active process of decision-making at all and inertia determines what happens next. It can be important to recognise that a decision to make no change, perhaps in the face of evidence that change is needed, is still a decision. Failure to listen to user demands for more appropriate services, for example, is a decision not to hear, just as surely as setting up an action group would be a decision to explore the potential for change.

However decisions are taken, conventional management literature recommends that they be based primarily on objective facts and figures. In social work, however, it is important to emphasise that values and assumptions always underlie the process. People's value orientations might be theoretical (for example, knowledge about child abuse might influence decisions about the allocation of resources); economic (deciding if costs outweigh benefits); aesthetic (appealing to personal preferences for order and attractiveness); social (placing value on the quality of human relationships); political (taking into account where power lies), ideological or religious (taking decisions according to beliefs about what is 'good' or 'right'). In management decisions, just as much as in practice, therefore, we need to be self-aware and able to analyse underlying agendas.

A normative or rational procedure for decision-making would take managers through the cycle of classifying and defining the problem or issue → developing criteria for a successful solution → determining the timescale and what process should be gone through, including how participative this can be in the time available → gathering all the necessary information → generating alternative solutions → comparing these potential solutions to the criteria, including by means of a cost–benefit analysis where necessary → selecting the most appropriate → implementing the decision → monitoring the implementation → evaluating the outcome(s). The resulting feedback would then be incorporated into any new definitions of the problem and so on round the cycle again. The process should always include time for reflection (what Pettinger, 1997, refers to as 'wait a minute'), so that the manager can consider any 'knock-on' effects, any implications for other individuals or groups of service users or staff, relevant aspects of agency policy and so on. It is easy to get 'bounced' into a decision by someone who asks 'It will be all right if I just do this, won't it . . .' and then to find that there are all sorts of unforeseen consequences.

The trouble with all decision-making models is that they tend to make it look as if the issue or problem is straightforward and not beset with conflicting needs or values. The real world of social work suggests that many decisions have to be made quickly, without all the information being to hand and often in an atmosphere of uncertainty. We need only consider the dynamics of decision-making in child protection cases to recognise how fraught the process can be. Management texts do recognise risk and uncertainty, and suggest minimising them by weighing up the relative impact of likely success and failure, involving those adversely affected in agreeing a way forward where possible (a care plan drawn up in partnership with parents; a redundancy package agreed with the workforce), and taking into account legislation and guidance, as well as the wider public interest (Pettinger, 1997). For larger scale decision-making, the manager may be assisted by public consultation, establishing a subcommittee or working group, or buying in consultants to produce a report outlining all the options and a recommended solution. It may be necessary to keep relevant groups briefed along the way and perhaps to ensure they receive support if the eventual decision is likely to lead to major life changes.

Where concentrated and perhaps collaborative thought is needed, an amazing variety of decision-making tools can assist (see Leigh, 1983), such as decision-tree analysis, brainstorming, the Delphi method and the nominal group technique, all of which are summarised below. Each of these is best suited to helping with one or more stages of the decision-making process so they can also be used in combination.

Superior decision-making might result from calling on the combined wisdom of a group. *Brainstorming* (see Figure 4.3) is an effective tool for creative problem identification. It involves a group of equal participants in face-to-face interaction, using free association of ideas to stimulate as many suggestions as possible. These are written down, as they come, without comment or discussion. The group then works together to draw out the common themes and explore any points that 'don't fit' in order to see whether they also need to be part of the picture. This can lead to reformulating the

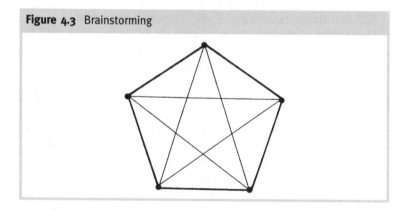

Figure 4.3 Brainstorming

problem. (These latter stages of the exercise are less well known than the first and are sometimes omitted, which simply results in an accumulation of free-floating suggestions that are not in usable form.)

Brainstorming can also be used to generate ideas on possible alternative solutions. A more sophisticated technique for thinking these through is *decision-tree analysis*, which is useful when a manager has to choose between different courses of action in a climate of uncertainty, where parts of the decision rely on chance factors or factors which lie beyond the manager's control. The 'decision tree' is so called because it resembles a tree (on its side). At any one time, two possible options represent branches off a larger trunk or branch, allowing a systematic appraisal of the opportunity that each branch represents and the likely consequences of choosing it. It is an incremental model, which allows each stage of decision-making over time to be plotted, illustrating the complexities of the choices involved and the reality of what is ruled in or out once one option has been selected. Bamford (1982) illustrates a decision of where to make budget cuts, which is shown in Figure 4.4.

The *Delphi method* (named after the Oracle at Delphi), unlike brainstorming, operates in an impersonal, anonymous setting in

Figure 4.4 A decision tree

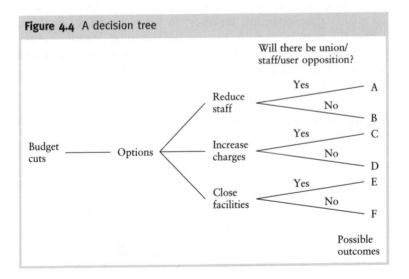

Figure 4.5 The Delphi method

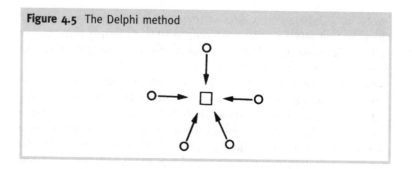

which opinions are voiced without bringing people together. The technique (see Figure 4.5) is really a way of collecting data from experts which is then coordinated through a central questioner (Bunning, 1979).

The *nominal group technique* is another creative procedure that combines the advantages of brainstorming and Delphi, using highly structured, face-to-face group meetings (Ford and Nemiroff, 1975). The group meets, but members generate ideas and alternative choices separately. It is an effective tool in reaching decisions, the group voting on the range of choices before them while a coordinator records the decisions, as shown in Figure 4.6.

It is acknowledged that, when a team participates, it gives everyone a sense of ownership in the eventual decision. We would want to qualify this statement, however, in the following cases. First, where the team lacks trust, motivation and good communication, and where destructive relationships and attempts to control one another exist, then the team leader may not get true participation.

Figure 4.6 Nominal group technique

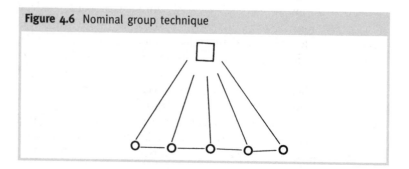

Second, the other side of the coin is where the group is excessively cohesive and rarely engages in conflict, so that poor decisions may result due to 'groupthink' (Janis, 1971). People in such groups are afraid to offer a different point of view and the team leader consequently may have to act as devil's advocate and stir up differences of opinion in order to stimulate reliable decisions.

As was noted above, decision-making is rarely as rational as the textbooks may suggest. Whatever decision-making method is chosen, there will inevitably be gaps in knowledge and a need to rely on best judgement. In the realities of policy and practice, compromises may be reached to save time or satisfy all those involved, or custom and practice may leave some options unexplored (Hill, 1997). The considerable dangers of this in high risk situations such as child protection or the care of vulnerable adults are obvious. The task of the manager is to ensure that there has been sufficient coverage of the relevant factors to provide an adequate evidence base for decisions reached.

Delegation

Delegating is sometimes awkward when assuming a managerial role for the first time; decisions have to be made whether to delegate upwards, downwards, outwards or to keep the work oneself. At the same time, the middle manager in particular has to keep an eye on the work that is sent her/his way. If asked to undertake duties that have little relevance to his or her role, these may have to be 'fielded' back.

Delegating too much or too little irritates one's colleagues. It can be the result of pressure or of not prioritising one's own workload demands. This may happen if staff get into a habit of pressurising the manager to do something immediately – taking the bait without giving oneself time to study whether the work is important will lead to poor decisions. When staff rush in and ask for a signature, it is usually sensible to require that the document be left for long enough to look it over. If we ourselves are unable to produce something immediately, we may send a 'holding' memo or a brief summary of where we are up to, just to give ourselves some breathing space and show that we have not forgotten the task. It is a sad fact that the more someone achieves, the more will be delegated their way; sometimes it pays to let people know how hard you are working, as well as with what good results.

The importance of delegating upwards merits emphasis; it is important to ensure that our own managers give us the support we need (and safeguard the organisation) by taking key decisions and reviewing potentially problematic issues. The consequences can be disastrous if senior management are not kept informed of any major concerns. Once they know that a problem is brewing, however, they can draw upon the whole range of managerial resources to deal with it, take legal advice if necessary and generally ensure that the middle manager does not feel alone in tackling something quite beyond his or her remit.

Delegating downwards relies on having a good knowledge of staff members, including level of competence, job description and current workload. It then involves weighing these against the task, the timescale and the standard to be achieved. In one sense, all management consists of delegation because the manager's role is to plan, coordinate and control the efforts of others. It is also sometimes necessary to identify someone to take on an additional task or responsibility. Already feeling uneasy at the first attempt at delegation of this kind, the new manager may find that it does not result in the person doing what has been asked. It is no use just giving someone a job and then leaving them to get on with it; this fails to indicate the time by which tasks have to be completed, it ignores the need to check that the duties are clearly understood and gives no scope for monitoring what progress is being made. It also overlooks potential resistance. It is necessary to be clear in saying what needs to be done and, if necessary, follow up a verbal request with a written memo. Also, when delegating a decision, it may be necessary to allow for the following:

● people have to work without interference (such as critical comments)
● usually there have to be incentives for the person doing the work, such as helping them build a CV or dropping another task to make space
● a delegated task must be accompanied by the time and resources to do it
● delegated decision-making requires equivalent delegated authority.

Although some of this takes more time initially, it is worth it in the longer term because it builds a team with whom the manager is able to share the work effectively. We have all known overworked managers who have failed to do this, at the expense of their own health and the well-being of their staff, not to mention the work the manager should actually be doing in planning and forecasting, organising and coordinating. It is also good for employees to develop their potential and become more involved in the agency's wider work. Satisfaction at work may be closely related to this kind of 'job enrichment' and opportunity for creativity.

Delegation always involves retaining oversight of the task or project in hand and requiring progress reports; it depends upon a combination of trust and control. At all times, the buck still stops with the manager, not with the staff member; anything else would be an abdication, not delegation, of responsibility (Pettinger, 1997).

Beyond leadership: the management of uncertainty

However good the manager, clear-cut decision-making depends on predictable circumstances and these simply do not pertain in social work any more. A new generation of thinkers have moved beyond classical management theory to engage with chaos theory and complexity theory (Haynes, 2003). Coming from the pure sciences initially, these are ideas that attempt to trace the order in apparent disorder and the potential for major impact of even the smallest change in a complex system. They recognise that simplistic notions of cause and effect may be outmoded and that, instead, it may be more fruitful to study critical incidents and risk factors at the local level. In this way, it is possible to engage with uncertainty by focusing on the particular interactions in the system that are most open to positive influence and most likely to prevent disaster. This has major implications for performance management approaches because the belief that outputs can be improved by controlling inputs across the board disappears as unworkably simplistic. On the other hand, it brings professional skill and judgement, and the creativity and flexibility long celebrated in social work, back to the fore.

Instead of seeing organisations as fixed and predictable entities, the newest approaches to management regard them as living systems (Geus, 1997). Because they are made up of human beings, they can adapt, change and self-organise. The behaviours involved are best understood through imagination and metaphor (Morgan,

1986, 1993). Management becomes a creative activity, able to cope with uncertainty and paradox, just as social work has always had to do. Learning to think, harnessing the unconscious mind and mental modelling all become better ways of coping with the human aspects of organisations than assuming that all decisions can be rational and all change predictable (Stacey, 2000).

Conclusion

To say that an organisation is well managed implies direction and intent, from the overall vision and purpose at the top, through strategic and operational planning in the middle, down to effective decision-making in well chaired meetings at team level. Equally, one should be able to see a line of communication and feedback going back the other way, so that senior managers are in touch with what matters to staff and service users. Responsibility for public money deserves no less and only in this way will responsive and effective services take the place of outmoded practices that have persisted by default. Over time, though, we have come to realise that management is often as much a creative as a rational activity – much like social work – and that the managers who can engage flexibly with uncertainty are perhaps nowadays the most likely to succeed.

In the personal social services, whatever their own style, even the best managers are only facilitators. It is a skilled and committed workforce which is the key to high quality services. Chapters 5 and 6 will look, first, at the recruitment and selection of staff and then at staff appraisal, development and care policies, all of which should combine into maximising what the human resource – the people employed there – can offer to a well managed organisation.

5 | Matching people and jobs

Nowhere is the tendency towards tighter management in contemporary social work more in evidence than in recruitment and selection. Consequently, this whole chapter owes as much to texts from human resource management (McKenna and Beech, 1995; Torrington and Hall, 1998), as to social work sources or the authors' own experience of appointing staff.

Until relatively recently, there were no particular difficulties in recruiting social workers – reflecting the job market, the age profile of the population and the fact that social work was not a regulated profession. The past ten years have seen a major change, marked by rising vacancy levels, heavy use of temporary staff supplied by employment agencies, increasing staff mobility and, consequently, significant challenges in recruiting and retaining staff at all levels. In such an environment, employers have to work far harder to attract staff and to encourage them to stay. This process starts with a positive recruitment process, meeting the interests of the potential employee as well as the needs of the employer.

Selecting the wrong person for a post has implications not only for that individual, but also for service users and future colleagues. It may also be damaging to the organisation if the ill-suited post holder goes on to make errors, upset valued staff or incur complaints. In the worst-case scenario, the considerable costs involved in disciplinary hearings, dismissal and renewed recruitment, even litigation, make improved selection procedures look cheap at the price. There are, of course, additional risks of attracting the wrong people into social work and hence further reasons for growing official interest in how staff are recruited (Warner, 1992; Support Force for Children's Residential Care, 1995; Kent, 1997). Direct access to children in some settings means that particularly careful screening of applicants and greater consistency between local authority employers are necessary. At the end of the day, all social workers are in positions of trust and have ample opportunities to exploit, rob or abuse vulnerable people.

To try and avoid mistakes, selection procedures have become more complex. There is a more managerial approach, with the emphasis on recruiting a flexible workforce to meet the organisation's constantly changing needs. To this end, a wider choice of *selection techniques* is deployed (with increased awareness of their respective strengths and weaknesses) and more use is made of outside agencies to recruit to top posts and temporary positions. At the same time, recruitment handled in-house may be used as an opportunity to promote the organisation's image to the outside world as clear in its direction, concerned for the people it serves and a good employer.

When a post falls vacant or is newly created, there are a number of tasks to perform. First, a job analysis is required, on the basis of which are prepared a job description, a person specification (outlining the essential and desirable requirements for the post) and the advertisement. (Job adverts are also used nowadays as an opportunity to present the organisation's corporate image to the outside world.) In some organisations, the human resources management (HRM, formerly known as 'personnel') staff undertake these tasks directly, in addition to their wider involvement in job evaluations, workforce planning, predicting the necessary skills mix, analysing turnover and so on. In others, the line manager or operational manager produces the documentation with backing from human resources to make sure that nothing contravenes industrial or discrimination legislation or agency policy, best practice is followed, and the highest calibre people are likely to be attracted without wasteful financial outlay. HRM staff are likely to deal with all the correspondence from enquirers and applicants, right through to formal notification of the outcome of selection, and to set up the shortlisting and selection procedures. We now look at each of the stages in turn.

Job analysis

Before a job description can be written, the *strategic needs of the organisation* have to be considered to ensure that this post, as currently designated, can be afforded and best meets the needs of the organisation, both now and in the foreseeable future. Once this thinking has taken place, a *detailed job analysis* can be prepared, listing the duties of the post. If a departing post holder is being replaced, it is clearly helpful to ask them, or someone doing an equivalent job, to outline:

- all the work activities involved, procedures followed and specific responsibilities
- whether the job requires any particular writing or computing skills, physical strengths or dexterity, or extensive reasoning and planning abilities
- whether detailed knowledge is required and, if so, in broadly what areas
- particular personal and interpersonal qualities needed, for example in working alone or in a team, or in building relationships
- working conditions, such as irregular hours or amount of travel involved.

The manager writing the analysis needs to work out whether any specific qualifications or experience are likely to be required for successful performance, and to check whether there are any agency policies on qualifications for this level of post.

In recent years, freezing vacant posts has been one of the few ways for social services to make sizeable savings. On a more optimistic note, we should remember that, with such a large proportion of the resources of a social work or social care agency tied up in its workforce, people leaving or retiring presents one of the rare opportunities to review how staff costs might be diverted into areas that are known to need expansion or updating. Or there may be other ways to get the same work done, for example through reorganisation, subcontracting, using the overtime budget or part-time staff or agency workers. Or it may be that the post can be retained but is in need of significant rethinking to ensure that it not only meets current demands but is flexible enough to anticipate future ones. Finally, there may be people who need to be absorbed into posts, rather than looking for people from outside, either as a result of internal restructuring or because a contract has been won to do work formerly undertaken elsewhere. This latter situation is dealt with by what are known as TUPE (pronounced 'chewpea') transfers under the Transfer of Undertakings (Protection of Employment) regulations.

Job description

Following on from the job analysis comes the job description: a concise summary of information about *what the post involves*. This comprises an outline of the job, the responsibilities involved, the competences and skills required in the post holder and the broad terms and conditions of employment. It will include the job title, grade (which may be flexible, depending on level of experience, skill and responsibility), location in the hierarchy, experience and professional qualifications required, hours to be worked and pay scale. It is a baseline for both the organisation (in selecting the best person and determining their rights to remuneration, training and so on) and the employee, for whom it constitutes a written statement of what they can expect and what is expected of them. In preparing it, care must be taken to observe relevant legislation and EU directives on matters such as the minimum wage and working time.

Usually accompanied these days by further particulars in an information pack, the job description itself includes a short paragraph giving the general 'feel' of the job. When it comes to specifics, it has become more common to place the emphasis on the competences the applicant will need and the management standards expected than on the detailed tasks he or she will be called upon to perform, because these tend to change so rapidly. Although the broad responsibilities of the post are still normally listed, it is also common practice to include a 'catch-all' clause at the end, such as 'any other duties as directed', so as to build in the possibility of *continuing development* and avoid a situation where the employee could later use the job description to pin down the employer and resist change when restructuring was planned. (The eventual employee may be required to sign to say that he or she has understood and accepted the job description, again to avoid objections at a later date.)

Some employers have gone further, following Japanese management practices, and have chosen not to specify which team the person appointed will be joining or what precise post they will take up. This gives the organisation the utmost flexibility in moving people around as required. A social work example of this is for a large employer to undertake mass interviewing in the early summer, when students are all emerging from local social work programmes, against vacancies which are bound to arise over ensuing months.

To sum up, a typical job description might include sections on:

- context of the job within the organisation
- job summary
- job content
- working conditions
- additional information
- the performance standards that the employer will expect, which, in social work, normally includes a commitment to equality.

Person specification

There are models available as to what kinds of things to cover in a person specification (Torrington and Hall, 1998, pp. 224–5). In social work, the emphasis is on qualifications, competences and aptitudes, relevant personal attributes and any special circumstances that may pertain (such as preparedness to work shifts or unsocial hours), rather than on general interests, personal presentation (although there may be a dress code for appearances in court, for example) or physique (unless there will be heavy lifting or other physical activity). It is important to ensure that nothing is included that cannot legally be justified in terms of anti-discrimination legislation. Disability discrimination legislation, for example, requires reasonable adjustments to be made to the pattern and place of work so that disabled applicants are not treated less favourably when being considered for jobs.

Against each of the headings selected as relevant, 'essential' and 'desirable' characteristics are listed. Like the job description, the person specification provides an important benchmark as to the qualities and qualifications the organisation needs and who should think about applying. Both shortlisting and interviewing are normally done against the person specification. Indeed, any major departure from it might give an unsuccessful candidate grounds to object. Where there is a surplus of candidates possessing all the essential characteristics, the desirable characteristics can be used to shortlist those who have more than the minimum to offer. It therefore makes great sense for applicants themselves to structure what they write around these characteristics, in order to help the selectors see precisely what they would bring to the post. This is especially helpful where there is a covering letter to write or a general section to complete and not just a straightforward application form to fill in.

Recruitment

Social work recruitment is usually done through newspapers and relevant professional journals, increasingly linked to websites. The advert normally only includes: brief details of the organisation; the job and duties; key points about the personnel specification, such as qualifications required (for example social work degree or equivalent); the salary scale; and how to apply.

Manual and clerical jobs are likely to be advertised in the local press and job centres, while professional and managerial jobs will appear in the social work and national press, with some employers feeling the need to use ever more eye-catching and upbeat advertisements to attract sufficient high quality applicants. It can be good for the employer and the profession to bring people in from outside, so as to spread fresh thinking and new practices. Internal applicants, on the other hand, offer the advantages of needing a shorter induction and, in the more senior posts, not having to be paid relocation expenses. Certainly, it is good anti-discriminatory employment practice to advertise all posts externally and it may also provide safeguards against the build-up of a negative culture – even an abusive network in residential settings – by ensuring that new and existing staff are not all previously known to each other or imbued with the same values (Levy and Kahan, 1991; Warner, 1992). Local authorities also use internal advertising, through intranet sites and noticeboards, in case there are staff who are looking for a change of responsibilities, working conditions (for example going part time) or location, whose needs can be met without being lost to the employer. In order not to discriminate indirectly against potential recruits from outside, however, this is typically combined with external advertising in some form.

Social work qualifying courses can have a positive effect on service delivery in their localities by attracting people from a distance, since, statistically, a high proportion of graduates settle in the area where they train. Providing placements for students is a good way of recruiting for social work organisations; employers have the opportunity to see the quality of students' work, evaluate their potential and attract them into jobs with the minimum of delay. It can therefore be seen as a useful investment of management time to work at ensuring sufficient practice learning opportunities to feed into the supply of high quality, new recruits.

Courses also attract local people who want to combine a good education with a vocational opportunity. Regions without a local higher educational institution or further education college offering diploma and degree-level qualifications may feel its lack, and employers have been known to work together to get a social work course set up nearby, sometimes as an offshoot of a more distant university. Over 90 per cent of those emerging from social work courses in the UK every year obtain social work posts within a relatively short time of graduating, giving social work education an exemplary employability record, as good as medicine, for example. Social work has been slow to link together workforce planning, on the one hand, and the location and size of social work courses, on the other. The government's concern about the recruitment and retention crisis in social work has led to central intervention in recent years to provide funding for a national recruitment campaign (www.socialworkcareers.co.uk), additional social work places in universities, bursaries at both undergraduate and postgraduate levels for those who study full time and traineeships in local authorities.

Social work has a reasonably good record in attracting students and employees from minority ethnic communities, but still more could be done. Vacancies do not yet appear routinely in the black press or get actively disseminated through informal communication networks such as noticeboards in relevant community centres. A wider issue here is the status and image of the profession of social work, which does not mark the pinnacle of 'making it' in Britain in the same way as becoming a doctor or a lawyer. When you add to this the fact that most people have relatively little idea what social workers actually do, there is a strong argument for publicising and promoting social work generally to whole communities and not just potential individual recruits through careers advice at school or in further or higher education. However, only jobs which are exempt from the provisions of sex discrimination or race relations legislation can actually specify, respectively, the gender or ethnicity of the person sought (see Chapter 7).

A greater number of disabled applicants may be attracted if proof is offered at this stage of a serious intention to adapt the working environment to their needs. For example, a minicom number can be provided for requesting application forms and these, in turn, can be made available in a range of communication formats.

Recruitment fairs or career conventions are now part of the national scene. They are attended by a combination of students in training, social work staff who may be thinking of changing employer and a general interest audience who may be considering a move into social work or social care as a career. A marked proportion of social work students are mature entrants who are making a career change. Again, this brings many strengths to the profession in terms of life and previous employment experience, whether in terms of another profession, such as teaching or the ministry, a previous job in a declining sector of heavy industry or a move from a less demanding and consequently unfulfilling job in another employment sector. Employers have also been bringing in qualified staff from overseas, notably from all parts of the English-speaking world such as Canada, Australia and New Zealand. Where the practice has involved deliberately tempting social workers away from countries with marked needs of their own, as in southern Africa, through the payment of an enhanced salary, this has been by no means uncontroversial.

Top management jobs are usually placed in the hands of executive search consultants ('headhunters'), whose task is to research the market, discover people who are doing well and are ready for promotion and encourage them to apply. They are often able to think laterally and consider fields in which people would have relevant skills and experience, without necessarily having worked their way up through the more obvious routes. This can be contentious if it leads to social work management posts being filled by non-social workers. Fair recruitment practices, especially in local government, always require openness and transparency, including opportunities for people to make a direct application alongside any search process that may be used, and for all those shortlisted to go through an interview process.

Shortlisting

Having advertised the post and, in most cases, attracted some interested applicants, the next decision concerns the selection of candidates for interview – shortlisting. Clearly, the people who do this should include those responsible for supervising the post and managing the service. The representativeness of the shortlisting panel (and the interviewing panel later on, which may well be bigger), for example in terms of gender and ethnicity, must also be taken into account.

The biggest variable in shortlisting is the total number of applicants; too few and it may be difficult to select high calibre staff, too many and a time-consuming and hence costly process ensues of attempting to construct a shortlist of manageable size. The emphasis (perhaps in the face of high levels of unemployment and hence heavy rates of applications in some employment sectors) has moved away from undertaking an initial screening to rule people out (which may allow arbitrary and perhaps unlawful criteria to creep in after the essential criteria have been met) and towards looking for the positive aspects, the strengths in each application that argue for that person to be included. Some big businesses are even using computers or automated multiple-choice telephone responses to pick out applicants who merit moving through to the next (human) stage of selection.

Once the essential points are covered, the criteria that were listed as 'desirable' may become crucial, as may other job-related issues, such as overall approach and vision and length and range of experience. A panel may each draw up a personal shortlist on this basis and then construct a final one, consisting of those applicants about whom everyone agrees and, if necessary, a sufficient number of others about whom consensus can be achieved. The only dangers are the inclusion of compromise candidates who offend no one but excite no one either, and the exclusion of maverick candidates, who approach a job in a way no one else had thought of but which may or may not be good for the organisation. A typical shortlist might consist of from three to six people, unless there is more than one vacancy to be filled. A good rule is to include no one on the shortlist who would not be really good in the post, that is, who is just 'making up the numbers'. Either the interview will waste their time and yours or, worse, they may end up as the compromise appointment, thus losing the real strengths that others could have offered, in one area if not in all.

Applicants for local authority posts are typically required to present themselves to the shortlisters through the medium of a printed application form with standard headings (although commerce has experimented with 'talking CVs', conveyed by digital camera and computer, and also personality tests conducted through the internet). Management trends in local government have meant that employers are keen to control the process of recruitment and selection, at the same time as streamlining it and saving time, by requesting information only as it relates to organisational needs. While the freestanding CV may give candidates scope to present themselves in their own terms, and show their abilities with computer presentation and writing skills, it is much more difficult for shortlisters to know whether the candidate had help with its production, perhaps even from a professional CV writer. Also, the only reliable way to obtain the same range of information from every applicant is to specify this in the application form, which then also becomes part of the record held by the employer on the individual eventually recruited. Obtaining information in a standard format and without gaps is also important, in respect of detecting those with a history of abuse (Support Force for Children's Residential Care, 1995) or if a 'biodata' approach is to be employed in systematically analysing all applicants (Audit Commission, 1995).

There are equal opportunities issues involved in aspects of the information which may be collected. Some potentially sensitive questions can be defended. Current salary is declared since the new employer would, in a normal career progression, usually be expected to match or better it. Any unexplained breaks in employment record could potentially relate to periods of mental ill health or imprisonment and will require clarification (Warner, 1992). All applicants must be asked to produce proof that they are entitled to work in the UK and should be offered the same list of alternative forms of documentary proof to establish this. Issues relating to gender, marital or parental status or ethnicity should *not* be enquired about in the form or the interview, as this poses a risk of racial or sex discrimination which are proscribed by statute. Similarly, the capacity of a disabled person to undertake a job must be seen within the context of what adjustments the employer can reasonably be expected to make to the working environment (see Chapter 7.) There may, quite properly, be a parallel process of equal opportunities monitoring, with separate, anonymised paperwork, which helps the organisation to evaluate the fairness of its employment practices over time.

Employers also now need to avoid discrimination on the grounds of age, religion or sexual orientation in employment, so that older workers, those of certain faiths and gay men and lesbians do not find themselves subjected to prejudices against which they have no redress. Managers must take care that panels avoid the widespread confusion between homosexuality and pædophilia, for example, making child care not the safest job in which to come out as gay. Naturally, this can pose a dilemma as to whether to declare oneself at interview and know where one stands, but risk not getting the job, or keep one's sexuality concealed and fear being outed at a later stage. The only way round this is for employers to make clear their stance on employing gay men and lesbians by incorporating it into their stated and published policy and ensuring that all interviewers are able to apply it fairly.

There is also a tension between gathering information that can help to identify those with a record of abuse (for example previous names) and that which might lead to discrimination, since reasons for changing one's name include religious and cultural affiliations and also gender reassignment (where gender history cannot legally be disclosed).

For disabled people, disability discrimination legislation now places the onus on the employer to take reasonable steps to adapt the workplace, through the provision of necessary facilities or support, or to alter current working practices so that potential disabled employees are not discriminated against (see Chapter 7). Examples of such adaptations might include providing minicom equipment to enable deaf employees to use the telephone (and, at the same time, ensuring that other relevant staff are trained to use it) or a scanner to transfer documents into Braille. It is important that individual needs are taken into account, however, since different equipment suits different people's needs. Shamefully, there are still constant reports that disabled people do not even get interviews for jobs for which they are eminently well qualified and that health and social care employers still tend to see disabled people as service users rather than potential colleagues. It is these attitudinal obstacles that will need to be overcome, along with the physical ones in the work setting. Now that the social model of disability is fundamental to social work service delivery, there is little excuse for it not to underpin employment practice in the same way and there is scope for this to receive far more discussion, both in management training and social work education, among the managers of tomorrow. Indeed, positive action can be taken, for example by shortlisting all disabled candidates who meet the essential criteria for the post.

In the meantime, shortlisters and selectors need to be sure that their own prejudices are not impinging on their decision-making, and training can help with this. This can apply to areas in which interviewers need to be more rigorous, as much as those where they may be blocking access to jobs unnecessarily. And, once a more diverse workforce has been recruited, there will be proportionately greater demands placed on the organisation's managers to manage diversity positively and creatively.

Selection

Selection is usually carried out on the combined basis of an interview, the application form and references, and perhaps psychometric or other forms of testing. Group selection methods are still found in social work education, because so much of the learning takes place in groups, and may be relevant for some work settings, such as group care. The more senior the post, the more complex and costly the process is likely to be, since the organisation wants to make sure of choosing the right person to cope with present-day demands. For example, there may be an additional element to the procedures if some particular presentational or other skills are involved in the job, for instance in a training post, which need to be tested on the day of the interviews.

Interviews

Interviews remain the most commonly used selection technique, despite frequently voiced doubts about their fairness or validity, that is, whether they are testing what they are intended to test or some other extraneous factors that creep into the process. Some of the doubts about interviewers' judgements include whether they are:

- too subjective
- based on initial surface impressions (favourable or unfavourable) of the interviewee's personal presentation or similarity in background to the interviewer, rather than on their ability to do the job

- further affected by these subjective or superficial impressions being communicated to the applicant early on in the interview, through tone or body language, so that he or she performs more or less well under their influence
- based around looking only for material to confirm a bias for or against the candidate, formed in the first few minutes of the interview or even before it, so that the interview becomes a self-fulfilling prophecy.

Clearly, these factors can combine together into an upward or downward spiral, working in favour of or against that particular candidate. Looked at more closely, all the problems listed lie more at the door of the interviewer than in the nature of an interview as such, which would suggest that there might be ways round them.

The first of these potential solutions, which is a norm in social work but not in all sectors of employment, is to have a *panel of interviewers* rather than a single person. Each may form a different impression of candidates that counterbalance one another, and particularly where the panel reflects the diversity of the community to be served by the person appointed. As with shortlisting, the make-up of the interviewing panel is important and should be based on anti-oppressive as well as HRM principles.

The involvement of service users in selecting the staff to work with them is increasing. This started in service provider settings, where those attending a centre or resident in an establishment either served on a selection panel or were formally involved in feeding in the collective views of users for the panel's consideration. Now, the involvement of service users is increasingly found in a range of appointments, up to and including directors of local authority services and organisations in the independent sector. Some senior managers have commented that their toughest interview was by service users, perhaps because users ask the blunt questions about where good quality services are going to come from and because they look for the people and the values behind the professional veneer (see, for example, Kahan, 1994, writing about young people). It is essential to have both clear guidance and required training sessions for *all* participants in the interview process, including service users. Furthermore, with panel members coming from widely diverse backgrounds, good chairing of both the interviews and the ensuing discussion is vital.

Second, training in selection and recruitment should encompass not only employment and anti-discriminatory legislation and best practice in human resource terms, but also the *interpersonal skills and awareness* involved in interviewing. Ideally, the opportunity to rehearse posing questions and listening attentively to the answers, and to see a playback of themselves on video, would help interviewers to overcome some of the pitfalls.

Appointments in some organisations involve local councillors, in local authority contexts, or board members or trustees in the independent sector, particularly at the more senior levels. There are numerous stories from earlier decades of such people favouring relatives or local constituents when making appointments, rather than appointing the best person for the job, or of them asking blatantly discriminatory questions. The more structured and regulated process that is now used, backed up by stronger equal opportunities and fair employment legislation, makes such malpractice less likely. Even so, the potential for tension between officers and elected members on interviewing panels in local authorities (or between paid staff and management board or committee members in the voluntary and private sectors) constitutes a strong argument for joint training. The widespread exposure of abusive practices in residential and other social care settings also stands as justification for the time and effort involved. Certainly, training for all selectors is recommended by the Audit Commission (1995), and training is equally important as a way of combating discrimination in selection practices (for example, CRE, 1993).

A well thought-out selection process will be designed to ensure that all candidates feel welcome and can give of their best, and that all members of the interview panel can participate effectively. It will entail, as a minimum, giving attention to all the following:

- the reception and waiting arrangements
- the layout of the interview room
- circulation of papers to all members of the panel well in advance
- providing them with a full briefing
- introducing the panel to the candidate and helping him or her to relax
- allowing uninterrupted and fair time with each candidate

- asking questions that are relevant to the job (and not other matters, such as family circumstances)
- ensuring that both questions and answers have been understood
- giving space for candidates to ask their own questions and add anything they feel the interview has not managed to glean about them that relates to their ability to do the job
- closing the interview smoothly and with mutual understanding about what will happen next
- making notes during or immediately after each interview, preferably on standard forms provided, which would stand up at a tribunal as providing sound reasons for the judgements reached. Time needs to be allowed in the interview schedule for this note-taking, as much as for interviews that overrun.

Disabled applicants should be asked if they need any particular provision in the interview, such as a sign language interpreter and/or information in an accessible format, and, of course, the venue should be fully accessible. Members of some social groups, who may have been disadvantaged in education (including disabled people and members of some minority ethnic groups), may have more to offer in life experience than in formal qualifications or may have had an unconventional career pattern. Depending on the demands of the job and the training opportunities available within it, there may be scope to consider any equivalence in particular strengths they might bring.

Equal opportunities interviewing

As one means of seeking to improve interviewing, in recent years local authority and other social work panels have often decided to ask the same questions of each candidate, based on the *key competences* involved in the job (together with reasons for wanting the post, for moving jobs at this time and so on), so that equality of opportunity is upheld. This procedure may even be organisational policy. At one time, this became an essentially mechanistic process, with each question asked, unembellished, like a mantra and with no follow-up. Yet the purpose of asking questions is presumably to find out more about the applicant's abilities and orientation to the post; this can scarcely be done if there is no content tailored to their particular circumstances or strengths.

Perhaps a useful distinction to be made is that between 'prompting' and 'probing'. Where one interviewee but not others is given prompts, or additional opportunities to go off in entirely new directions at the whim of the selector, this can be seen to be unfair. Where, however, further probing questions are asked, on the basis of what each person has already said or has written on their application, they are merely being allowed to do themselves justice in responding to the set questions, provided that this happens for all those seen and does not become too personally intrusive. Areas that will certainly need to be probed include any gaps in employment history and any concerns raised by the application or references. Where a candidate has had personal experience of abuse or other trauma, this could give them a great empathy with service users but it may be important to be clear that they are at a stage of readiness to help others (Barter, 1997), perhaps through conducting a preliminary interview under equal opportunities conditions (Warner, 1992). More generally, attitudes to power and authority, and to sexuality and other sensitive issues, should arguably be gauged for all candidates for posts in residential child care (Kent, 1997).

Furthermore, the quest for complete uniformity in interview procedure was arguably bound to fail. A selection panel might unwittingly influence the outcome in any number of ways: the skill with which applicants are settled down in the interview room; the tone in which questions are posed; the sequence in which people are interviewed (for example because of the degree of attentiveness from a panel that is ready for its lunch or drowsy afterwards); and so on. Even if some device like interviewing in alphabetical order is decided upon, where a good applicant follows a poorer (or poorly interviewed) one, or vice versa, the 'contrast effect' can come into play so that perspective is lost on their actual performance (Anderson, 1985). Nevertheless, the happy medium is certainly to retain some overall structure because it can be explained to candidates, facilitates comparisons between them and makes it easier to keep notes. The panel chair should ensure that decisions, and the grounds on which they were reached, are systematically recorded as a defence against any later challenge of unfair treatment and for evaluation purposes.

For those who wish to pursue their reading in this area, particularly in the context of formal study, there has been some complex theorising about the dynamics of interviewing and the problems inherent within it. A Foucauldian analysis of the power relations in human resource management and the discourses operating within it, for example, is offered by Townley (1994).

Other approaches to standardised interviewing

Other employment sectors, notably business, have experimented with different ways of trying to standardise interviews and tie them more closely to the matters they are supposed to be testing. These include *situational* or *critical incident interviewing*, based around asking how applicants would cope with particular situations that might crop up in the job (the job analysis can help to identify these), and the *patterned behaviour description interview*, which probes a series of major life changes to try and identify whether there is a pattern in the way the candidate deals with problems and challenges. Both these approaches may tend to assume that there is one optimal way of reacting and that the panel knows what it is. Nevertheless, they are not entirely foreign to ideas that can be found in theorising social work intervention, they do attempt to stick to matters related to carrying out the job, and they may produce more valid and standardised results than less structured methods that leave the candidates free to talk about whatever they consider relevant in response to each broad question.

A final method that may resonate even more closely with current social work thinking is *competency-based interviewing* (Johnstone, 1995). Here, the focus moves from what candidates have achieved to how they achieved it, so as to identify the skills or traits that underpinned their achievements. Once again, the questioning starts from specific situations, this time in previous employment experience and asks what were the tasks, the actions and the results that ensued. This gives the acronym STARs: or Situations, Tasks, Actions, Results.

Whether or not one of these more structured methods of interviewing is followed, it is generally more productive to pose a hypothetical situation, or ask the interviewee to tell you about a specific experience in their area of practice, than to ask closed questions with 'yes/no' answers. Asking someone whether they agree with anti-racist policies, for example, is of little help since they can hardly say they don't. Asking them to describe one occasion when these policies have created opportunities or challenges in their working life and what they did about it will be far more revealing.

Participative interviewing

Despite the inevitable pressures, a job interview should be an opportunity for *two-way communication* and, although there is less likely to be the hard bargaining over pay and conditions in social work that is seen in business circles, the applicant does need the chance to check on issues that may be unclear or of particular personal importance and perhaps to make certain requirements clear. More than this, he or she should be given the opportunity to be actively engaged in the recruitment and selection process by being valued and listened to at all stages. A profession such as social work that prides itself on partnership should surely be keen to support this more reciprocal approach to selection, and not one that is based on assuming that 'management knows best'. At the end of the day, in hearing fully from candidates what they have to offer, we can show that we are 'concerned not only with the job to be done, but also with the work that is offered' (Torrington and Hall, 1998, p. 222). The more information candidates have had about the job, the more there can be an element of *self-assessment* in what they write and say about their ability to do it.

When the panel comes to consider its decision, it may also take into account any feedback from the team the candidate would be joining, if a meeting with, or presentation to, its members constituted part of the selection process. After all, they are the people who will be working with the successful applicant and they are among the ones who will suffer most directly if a misjudgement occurs in selection. Care must be taken, however, that all candidates have an equal chance to present themselves to the team, and that feedback about the team's views is sought systematically on each, in order to avoid introducing unequal treatment into the process at this point. Involving prospective colleagues in this way also means that unsuccessful candidates for the post are not able to keep the matter confidential. It may therefore be sensible to advise the wider team, as well as the interview panel, about appropriate protocol.

Police and other checks on suitability

The panel must be informed of the outcome of police checks for many social services posts with direct contact with the public. Child sex abusers may actively target residential child care and daycare settings (Kendrick, 1997; Colton and Vanstone, 1998) and wholly unsuitable people may also be attracted to working with other vulnerable groups. There are no certain ways of identifying abusers in advance, but checking with the national Criminal Records Bureau (in Scotland, the Scottish Criminal Records Office) will at least reveal whether the individual has any relevant convictions or cautions, including any offences of violence or dishonesty, as will a check against the register of convicted sex offenders. Part 2 of the Criminal Justice and Court Services Act 2000 allows an order to be imposed, banning from either paid or unpaid work with children anyone who has committed a serious offence against a child (www.homeoffice.gov.uk/cjcsguide.htm). Such offences now include having abused a position of trust by having a sexual relationship with a 16- or 17-year-old in care or detention. Furthermore, there is a central access point (List 99) for information about those banned by the Secretary of State for Health from working with children, whether in a paid or unpaid capacity (and an index for this purpose in Scotland; see Scottish Office, 1998).

Although police checks can take some weeks to come through, an appointment should not be confirmed until this happens, or, at least, the appointee should not work unsupervised with children or vulnerable adults in the interim. For social work posts, it should be noted that convictions do not become 'spent' under the Rehabilitation of Offenders Act 1974, meaning that the offences can be taken into account for life.

An additional safeguard is provided, in the form of a register of all qualified social workers and social care staff. Employers are required to consult with the register when making new appointments. Registered individuals who are found guilty of unprofessional conduct may, in serious cases, be struck off, preventing them from working in the field in the future. The names of those struck off will be available to employers to prevent re-employment by another organisation. The GSCC will itself be able to consider cases of professional misconduct that do not result in criminal proceedings, which should put an end to most cases of abusers moving around to avoid disciplinary action by any one employer.

The system is not problem-free, either as regards safeguarding children or in respect of the civil liberties of job applicants. The free movement of workers within the EU is a matter of some concern, for example, because of the complexities it introduces into the checking procedures. Recruitment overseas may pose similar challenges.

There may, in effect, be no way of obtaining sufficiently detailed information from the other country or countries where the applicant may have worked, and not every state has reached the UK's level of awareness of the dangers of child abuse. Thinking about the individual applicant, on the other hand, the police checks that are made here not only produce hard data on criminal convictions but also 'soft' information held by the police which might relate to more general concerns or a possibly disguised identity. One of the authors has had experience of several worrying examples of details sent through by the police, including a lesbian student who felt she had been unfairly targeted by the police in a series of incidents that were now recorded on the police computer, and an Asian student with a common name, which, when entered into the police computer, elicited confidential information about several other people of a similar age living nearby! Clearly, we would want to know about anyone who, although not actually convicted of an offence against children, had already given rise to serious concerns but, in an over-eagerness to try and protect the public, there could be serious injustice or an infringement of liberty. Social workers are used to seeking a balance between individual and group rights – this is an area in which the reality comes close to home. On balance, it is better for the public and the profession for there to be a clear process to identify the risk of abuse and to do all that is possible to prevent it. Within this, it is essential that people can challenge and defend themselves against mistaken allegations, and that the system is open, transparent and seen to rely on evidence rather than rumour. Identity theft poses a further challenge to keeping track of applicants' backgrounds.

Even with a robust system in place, a further concern is the possible lack of consistency with which interview panels and employing organisations act on police or other relevant information once they have received it. In one research study, for example, a hypothetical interview exercise led to a fictional candidate, described as having quite a serious conviction for an offence against a child, being considered by some people as appointable to a post with direct access to children (Smith, 1999). The people concerned, although role-playing in the exercise, were making the same type of judgement as they were called on to exercise in their actual jobs. There is no way of knowing how often this kind of laxity may be occurring in real life. Given the scandals in a number of residential child care settings (see, for example, Williams and McCreadie, 1982; Hughes, 1986; Levy and Kahan, 1991; Jones, 1996), it is vital that the channels government has given the profession (and which the profession long requested) to regulate and monitor its workforce be utilised according to appropriate conduct and practice standards. Otherwise, all the official reports and reviews, for example those that made relevant recommendations to try and protect children in residential care (Utting, 1987, 1997; Skinner, 1992; Warner, 1992; Support Force for Children's Residential Care, 1995; Kent, 1997), will have been in vain.

The use of tests in selection

Psychological testing

Psychological or psychometric testing has been growing in favour among social work employers, again as a reaction against the subjectivity of interviewing. Tests in use in social work contexts are more likely to be designed to gauge personality than general intelligence (as defined by test designers). They include some that have been devised to test the suitability of candidates applying to work with children and even their potential to abuse. Since most of the abuser population is hidden and since abuse is rooted in denial and minimisation, even to the self, it is hard to see how such tests have been standardised, although they claim high levels of validity. Nevertheless, it is understandable that employers would want to do everything possible to avoid placing trust in a likely abuser and recent government-backed advice is that such tests, provided they are professionally assessed, may have a useful role to play (Support Force for Children's Residential Care, 1995; Kent, 1997).

Like interviews, tests do not always measure what they are meant to measure. Just as IQ testing has long been known to involve many elements of motivation and performance in a test situation, over and above the content of the test itself (and this has been suggested as one reason why some ethnic groups perform better than others), criticisms of psychometric testing include an accusation that they have been designed around white norms and that African-Caribbean candidates may do less well and hence lose out on being appointed to posts for which they are perfectly well suited (Skellington with Morris, 1992). This also begs the wider question as to whether candidates must always be fitted for jobs or whether jobs might sometimes be adapted to benefit from the skills of less traditional candidates.

Furthermore, the tests are useful only if they can be shown to relate to the skills and qualities actually involved in doing the job *and* if there is agreement as to which are the most advantageous of these. As we saw in Chapter 2, there is a strong move in some management quarters away from macho management and towards networking and teamwork. Thus the 'right' answers to a leadership test last week might be the wrong answers this week. And the job itself might change quite radically over time.

At the extreme, no organisation desires an emotionally unstable workforce and motivation can certainly be considered more relevant to employment contexts than it is to measures of intelligence. So tests may not be all bad. Nevertheless, the other aspects of personality that tests purport to measure (risk-taking or playing safe, being controlling or submissive and other areas of strength and confidence) might arguably be needed in some degree of balance within a team. A children's home might be an equally untherapeutic place if all the staff were trying new ideas all the time as if no one was. And no team can survive if everyone is trying to lead it. The aim of the psychologists in creating a standard profile for each job may therefore be an essentially unhelpful one in social work.

Test designers themselves own up to certain flaws in the notion of testing, such as the chance of people giving dishonest or only socially acceptable answers. They attempt to build in safeguards so that other psychologists will accept them as valid (actually testing what they set out to test) and reliable (producing comparable results over time). Social scientists in other fields may draw a distinction between people's answers to hypothetical questions and what they do in real life, or may see human beings as a complex combination of characteristics affected by context and interactions with others, rather than as a series of 'types' that can be neatly labelled and measured. We would all like to think that we know ourselves, and most of us love to score ourselves in magazine quizzes, but, faced with an emergency or a true test of leadership, we very often do not know exactly what strength of courage, resilience or resourcefulness we would find. The best test, probably, is how we have behaved in any similar circumstances in the past and we have already seen how an interview can focus on that.

Nevertheless, the use of psychometric tests as one part of the selection process is growing, especially among large organisations and for more senior posts. It is therefore important to remember that the testing is not an objective, scientific solution to the vagaries of interviewing but actually has some of the same weaknesses built in. Even where properly qualified testers are paid large sums to undertake it, they are subject to the same difficulty in getting the organisation to specify exactly what it is looking for, the same challenge in really knowing how to match an infinite variety of human beings to the narrow constraints of paid employment and the same artificiality built into the whole selection process. There remain many aspects of individuals that tests cannot measure and the data they produce should always be incorporated carefully into the more wide-ranging information gathered by other means.

Work-based tests

A different sort of test that may be combined with an interview is the *work-based* or *in-tray* test. This may give the candidate a representative sample of work to do, possibly complete with interruptions and emergencies, and ask how they would prioritise it and what tasks they would carry out, or it may be based around one case study in which a decision or a care plan is needed. This technique has certainly been used in social work selection.

While closer to the 'real world' than psychometric testing, it is still devoid of context, and also subject to the candidate's interview nerves and other drawbacks of the artificiality of the situation. Always assuming that the selectors are skilled enough not to look for 'right answers' but viable and professionally justifiable ones, there is still the issue of how they can use this one-off technique to evaluate what a candidate would be bringing to a job that may change considerably over time and in which the contribution of some intangible flair or vision might be advantageous. Nevertheless, this may be the closest social work practice can get (because it tests practice skills) to the almost universal requirement in education and training for applicants to demonstrate their practical teaching skills through a presentation to their potential colleagues.

Presentations can also explore a candidate's knowledge of policy and practice agendas, and ability to project ideas and personal vision for the organisation; hence they are widely used for management-level posts. Certainly, there needs to be some attempt to evaluate the skills the candidate would actually use in the job if we are to avoid the 'Peter Principle' (Peter, 1970), whereby people are promoted to the level of their own incompetence, that is, to the job above that in which they have already demonstrated they can cope (or at least avoid doing any real harm). Those who will make the best managers may not be those who made the best social workers, therefore the profession may gain an inadequate manager at the expense of a competent practitioner.

Aptitude tests

Where the employee will be called on to exercise particular practical skills such as word processing or desk-top publishing, there is every reason to set a pre-interview exercise that tests these quite specifically and can be incorporated into selection decisions.

References

In a profession like social work, references about past job performance and general good character are clearly essential. They should be derived from professional sources who have known the candidate in a previous professional or caring role, including the current or most recent employer, and should be conveyed direct to the recruiting organisation, not via the candidate so that there can be no question of forgery or tampering.

Each agency has its own policy regarding when selectors should read references, either before or after the interview. If taken up in advance, then any negative or unclear points from the references may be explored in the interview. References have, however, tended to become ever more bland since there have been legal challenges to their contents (which, if defamatory, can unfairly cost someone the job), and it can take a great deal of reading between the lines to spot any dissatisfaction or unease. On the other hand, in social work, a future employer or service user could equally well have a case for damages against a referee who had failed to reveal adverse information about an applicant from which some harm later resulted (Warner, 1992).

The main function of a reference is probably to verify that the applicant has the employment record they claim, and has not done anything in a recent post that has resulted in disciplinary action or other formally recorded outcome that has given rise to concern. Thus, the reference is often made a condition of appointment, rather than a tool to assist the interviewers, and reading it may be left until after the candidate is seen so as not to bias the process. This can be frustrating for the reference writer who takes care to express both the strengths and weaknesses they feel should influence the matching of candidate to job, for example a need for support or a protected caseload in a first post or a more developed level of skill in one type of practice than another. Practice may swing back towards reading references in advance in the light of views taken in the residential child care field, where it is increasingly felt that concerns should be probed in the interview rather than risk giving candidates the benefit of the doubt (Warner, 1992; Support Force for Children's Residential Care, 1995; Kent, 1997). Also frustrating for the conscientious referee is the trend towards 'tick box' references, which seek to gauge the candidate's level of competence without offering the writer any chance to 'bring the person alive', although they are certainly quicker to complete and ensure that standard information is provided.

From the applicant's point of view, of course, it can be a worry to have one's future fate controlled by a current employer, tutor or practice teacher. There are many stories of managers who are said to write bad references for staff they want to retain, sometimes in jobs and at salary levels that vastly undervalue their potential, or of whom they are jealous or resentful. Certainly, any applicant should have the right not to have their present employer consulted for a reference until a late stage in the process. This is partly because it may be awkward to let the employer know that another post is being considered and the individual may fear that annoying their current manager could affect not only the outcome of their application, but also the way they might be treated in their current workplace afterwards. Or, where the job seeker is a manager, having the team knowing that he or she is on the lookout for another post can have a destabilising effect, or can lead to jockeying for position as people wonder who will get the soon-to-be vacant job. Conversely, there are some employment contexts where an employee who is known to have been shortlisted for another job is more likely to be retained through internal promotion or other recognition. Much depends on the culture of the organisation and the perceived value of the particular staff member in terms of skills and experience.

Just as with job applications, the advent of human resources

managers in social services has brought with it standardised reference forms designed to mirror the competences and qualities
required in the job and key aspects of what is known of the applicant from his or her last work setting. His or her sickness record
increasingly features, alongside confirmation of post held, dates
employed, nature of the referee's relationship with the applicant,
for example line manager, university tutor, how long they have
known one another and so on. Given the nature of social work,
there cannot help but be an element of the character reference, in
that any information that may be known regarding criminal record
or unprofessional conduct ought to be declared. A fuller reference
will talk about the candidate's performance in their last job or on
their qualifying programme. Although the applicant nominates
their own referees, there is an almost unvarying requirement in
social work to have the last employer nominated and some agencies
are very particular about the management level at which the reference can be signed. This is intended to ensure that the next
employer is not falsely reassured about someone who has actually
not been trustworthy in holding social work responsibilities.

It is the norm in the UK to require references and, far from
falling from favour as low on validity, they are being standardised
for management credibility along with every other aspect of the
recruitment and selection procedure. Indeed, referees may be
approached by telephone in relation to residential child care posts
to ensure that they have had the opportunity to comment frankly
on what they have written about the candidate's strengths and
weaknesses (Kent, 1997; Utting, 1997). Once again, a potential
tension can be perceived here between users' rights (in this case
children's rights) and equal opportunities in the workplace, since it
might be far more difficult to challenge something afterwards that
had been suggested over the phone rather than written down in a
reference. At the very least, applicants should be told that the
employer reserves the right to contact any previous employer. This
can carry risks, though, in that there has been an out-of-court
settlement and also an adverse local government ombudsman
judgement concerning information on a reinstated employee and a
withdrawn allegation passed, in each case, from a current to a
prospective employer and later deemed confidential (*Community
Care*, 16–22 September 1999, pp. 6, 12). The same debates apply
to whether written references should be confidential or open.

Currently, referees are often given the choice, open references having formed part of a wider trend towards freedom of information, but there may be some evidence of a swing back to confidentiality as more likely to lead to a frank sharing of concerns (Kent, 1997).

Other outside information about the candidate which may be taken into account is a medical report which states whether their physical condition is considered suitable for the job and a declaration by the candidate of any previous criminal convictions or cautions, which would be followed up. Also, since it is now the employer's legal responsibility to establish the right to work in the UK, all candidates are now asked to produce documentary evidence that they possess this right. In order to avoid discrimination, it is important that all are presented with the same choice of documents that will suffice – not passports for minority ethnic candidates and evidence of National Insurance status for others, to take a worst-case scenario. It is also a sensible precaution to check professional qualifications with the awarding body and ask for proof of the applicant's current address.

Feedback to candidates

Organisations vary in whether or not they give feedback to unsuccessful candidates. In the main, it is considered useful for people to be given constructive comments on how they came across and advice on how they might enhance qualifications, experience and so on. On the other hand, there is a constant fear in these litigious days of challenge through employment tribunal, and employers may fear giving opinions that could be actionable. Verbal rather than written feedback, based on agreed interview notes, may be a partial protection.

Internal candidates

Once a job is advertised, then staff within the organisation may apply. This can create dilemmas for the manager if an internal candidate is not appointed, especially if that person has been acting up in that post for some time, because it can, although not inevitably, lead to lowered morale and commitment. Keeping a valued member of the team is possible not only through promotion but by ensuring that their workload is sufficiently challenging and rewarding. Just as much stress occurs with underwork as overwork, so such a person might be asked if there were tasks they would wish to develop so that everyone could benefit from fresh insights and ideas. If the internal candidate is successful, it is vital that their existing commitments are taken from them; it is not uncommon for staff to be expected to cope, at least in the transition period, with two jobs.

Monitoring and evaluation of selection

Like any other aspect of the agency's work, selection should ideally be monitored and evaluated over time. This can include: asking both the selectors and the candidates to fill in a brief questionnaire about the process and whether it enabled the candidate to perform optimally and helped the selectors to obtain the information they needed about both the vacancy and the candidates; monitoring the progress of newly appointed candidates to ascertain whether they perform to the level expected; and comparing different selection methods to gauge which appear to have the greatest validity. Adverts can also be monitored to find out which were the most effective in attracting high calibre candidates.

Induction and departure: rites of passage

Two phases of working life sometimes ignored in management literature are those of orienting a new member of staff and saying goodbye to one who is leaving. When planning an induction programme, the manager will need to decide which areas of information can be left to the headquarters system to deliver and which are better handled by the team. Usually, others explain the organisational structure, where the person fits into it and what the regulations are (for instance in relation to health and safety). It is helpful for the team leader to spend some time with the new worker, possibly giving a brief history of the team, its philosophy, how the workload might be reallocated to fit with what the person can offer, and perhaps explaining procedures. Any adaptations that a disabled inductee may need should be finalised at this time.

Too much information at this stage could be confusing and so the team leader might link the new member with close colleagues or an experienced member of staff as a mentor for a short period. Introductions to key figures and resources can be undertaken by this colleague. Staff in group care are typically 'thrown in at the deep end'; whether or not this happens or if, in fieldwork, a ready-made caseload is waiting, immediate exposure is not necessarily harmful provided that there is a supportive climate in the establishment. What is unhelpful is seeing induction as a once-and-for-all event: a person's passage into an organisation has to be planned on an unfolding basis, where there is scope to learn and develop throughout one's career. It is also a two-way process. The organisation needs to set some parameters about expected standards of behaviour, familiarise the individual with their new job and working environment and offer any necessary training, for example in using the in-house computerised recording system, but it is also important to hear from them what they need to know in the early stages and how they learn most effectively. Any manager who has previously been a practice teacher will have developed useful skills in helping people to settle in. It is also useful to remember that there is an informal as well as a formal side to induction. People form personal impressions from the way they are treated (at selection and after), from things they have read or heard about the organisation and sometimes from past dealings with it. The formal induction may need to correct some of these impressions (Pettinger, 1997).

At the opposite end of a career, when an employee is leaving, the manager's sensitivity is similarly essential; a sense of loss generally accompanies each leaving, so a lunch or a gift tends to mark the occasion. Often, people are leaving to begin a new stage in their life, which can be celebrated with them in a way which recognises that we do all have lives beyond the job and have valued one another's support and company as people, not just as colleagues. Even with an unsuitable worker, there will have been some professional and personal strengths which can be acknowledged, so that positive factors are to the fore at the point of leaving.

But where an employee is suspended or summarily dismissed for misconduct (see also Chapter 4), there may be an embargo on others speaking to them outside the formal procedures, which can make it impossible to do the human things one would naturally want to do. Sometimes the person becomes so angry that even a neutral enquiry as to how they are coping might be misconstrued, or they are so upset that any such enquiry is turned into an inappropriate conversation about all that has happened. It is at times like this that other support structures such as trade unions and staff care services come into their own and it is usually advisable to leave them to support the individual who is being investigated. At the end of the day, the first responsibility of other employees is to the general public, including service users. This must outweigh allegiance to a colleague and perhaps friend, who is thought not to have upheld the standards those services demand or has shown in some other sphere of life that they cannot be trusted (not to be violent or dishonest, for example). Having said that, it is recognised that any suspension causes great pressure for the person under investigation and the others around them (including any who may be called as witnesses), all of whom will need support, and that it is potentially divisive for the team. Conflict resolution at an early stage or mediation through the BASW Advice and Representation Service or through ACAS would be a positive step, if appropriate, although sometimes matters have already gone too far or the alleged misconduct is simply too grave (Dadswell, 1999).

Fortunately, many potential problems with employees can be avoided by adequate staff development – with appraisal mechanisms and training opportunities feeding positively into one another (see Chapter 6) – and by the provision of timely advice through guidance or warnings, incorporating stated targets and timescales for improvement. Above all, clearly stated performance standards and agency policies and protocols mean that there can be no doubt what is expected, although they do risk making social work practice more mechanistic and rigid than it used to be. And all disciplinary matters must be dealt with fairly, giving the individual a right to a hearing, consistent treatment, an unbiased decision with stated reasons and provision for appeal. These 'procedural rights' are the cornerstone of an individual's civil rights, in employment as elsewhere (Galligan, 1992).

Conclusion

We have seen in this chapter how managerialism in social work has made its mark on the recruitment and selection process and also how (post)modern organisations deliberately recruit for a climate of flexibility and change. The workforce that is faced with these imperatives is bound to experience an increased level of job demands and pressures, which, in turn, makes staff development and staff care policies all the more important. We will examine these in Chapter 6.

6 | The human resource: meeting the needs of staff

The largest element of the budget in human service organisations is spent on salaries: the 'human resource' – a huge step forward from the early 'cogs in a machine' thinking noted in Chapter 2.

An organisation's employees are a major asset, not only in themselves, but also because the organisation's whole reputation and future success depend on them. Consequently, it is a false saving to skimp on staff support or development. These are arguably the most direct ways to influence the quality of organisational performance as well as retaining and fostering the best employees. It is better value to invest in a workforce than constantly recruit and train replacements, most notably recognised in the Investors in People scheme (http://www.investorsinpeople.co.uk) to which many local authorities have subscribed.

As befits husbanding a precious resource, 'getting the best out of staff' is a concern for the whole organisation, not just the line manager. Good supervision combines management, education and support (see www.doh.gov.uk/pdfs/stand15.pdf). The organisation needs frameworks that encompass these three elements which, on this larger scale, become performance appraisal, staff development and staff care.

Supervision

In these managerialist days of targets and measurement, one of the great dangers is that the need for personal discussion is lost in an obsession with data. There can be no substitute for talking on a regular basis about developments in individual cases and a good supervisor will be able to bring together the performance data and the experience of the social worker to make a coherent whole. In the best organisations, this is empowering for staff, productive for the organisation and beneficial for service users.

Supervision continues to serve several purposes at once and some accounts tend to present this as a problem. Lishman (1998, p. 98), for example, sees competing claims as a 'potential dilemma and danger' and Turner (1995, p. 127) as a subversion of professional development into 'a means of controlling or instructing staff'. It is certainly true that these functions have to be held in tension, with the achievement of stated outcomes now essential in all spheres of work, but it could equally be seen as a remarkable achievement that our profession has so tidily combined several different complex requirements into one process, with such economy of time and effort. Few work settings can claim a mechanism which, at its best, so smoothly combines the oversight of work undertaken, performance, developmental and staff care considerations.

Because it is the norm in social work to combine these functions, the biggest shift for the newly promoted manager is in having to face in two directions at once – towards the staff they are supervising (to meet their support and development needs and help them exercise judgement wisely in their assessments and interventions) and towards their own managers (to meet the needs of the organisation in getting the work done appropriately).

Becoming a supervisor for the first time can be daunting. When one of the present authors was first promoted, an experienced manager commented: 'Now you will find that your staff cause you more problems than service users ever did!' It is all too easy to feel that experienced staff are more skilled than you are or the newly qualified more 'up' on the new ideas, that you have not been trained in professional supervision, that staff see what you offer as merely checking up on them, or to ask why you should bother to supervise others when you yourself do not receive adequate support or advice. In some places, supervision is still associated with merely checking that procedures are complied with and expenditure accounted for, so that frontline managers may find that their job lies mainly in gathering management information and balancing budgets.

However, supervision has become the focus of renewed interest and is now recognised in government guidance as the bedrock of safe and effective services (see, for example, www.doh.gov.uk/pdfs/stand15.pdf). The crisis in social work recruitment and retention has drawn attention to the need to spend time on supporting and encouraging individual staff, whether new to the organisation or of longer standing. In the wider society, across all sectors, supervision is seen as vital to performance management, staff development and business success, reflected, for example, in the Investors in People standards.

One of the greatest joys of any manager's work is to foster the skills and talents of others, to see people achieving their full potential and flourishing over time and to assist them in giving a good professional service to others. Sometimes all it takes to do this is a listening ear, a few questions to draw them out, some words of praise or guidance, and ensuring that you yourself keep on top of what is happening in the wider agency and, preferably, in the profession as a whole. More positive trends that may support managers in offering supervision include 'reflective practice' (see below), which relies on practitioners being given opportunities to stand back and question their approach to their work, and a project at NISW on the 'management of practice', which demonstrated that supervision needs to go beyond checking up on managerial objectives into supporting individuals in developing better practice (Kearney, 1999). This also resonates with the constant calls in inspection reports for higher standards of supervision.

An organisation that can 'grow its own' (develop and promote its own staff) can minimise recruitment problems and bolster standards. So the new manager can fairly make demands for training in how to supervise and for help with meshing supervision into broader agency strategy. He or she can also reasonably ask staff to be well prepared and to work at getting the most out of supervision (Knapham and Morrison, 1998).

Purpose of supervision

The overall purpose of supervision must be to enhance the standard of work undertaken so that, in turn, vulnerable members of the public will have an improved quality of life. To do this effectively, while also ensuring that the person being supervised is able to make the most of the opportunity, supervision should be grounded in the principles of anti-oppressive and best practice.

More specifically, supervision is intended to:

● **Meet managerial and administrative needs by:**
   – assisting with workload management, for example reviewing and planning work
   – monitoring day-to-day work to ensure that it is carried out well and within agency policies and priorities

  - providing a sounding board for ideas, concerns, plans and strategies
  - keeping the staff member in touch with developments in resources, statutory requirements, departmental policies and so on, and the ways these relate to his or her work
  - giving feedback about performance
  - ensuring that manual or computerised recording is of the required standard and up to date
  - providing the supervisor with part of the management information needed to keep an oversight of the throughput of work in the team and the rate of resource allocation to carry out that work.
- **Meet educational and developmental needs by:**
  - promoting professional and personal development
  - providing learning opportunities to keep knowledge and skills up to date
  - developing awareness of role and responsibilities within the organisational context
  - helping the worker acquire greater understanding of people, problems and situations
  - building professional confidence, creativity and new ways of working.
- **Meet support needs by:**
  - providing emotional support, for example helping someone rediscover the rewards in their work where motivation has flagged, reviewing an overload of work, providing new challenges so that staff continue to grow in their jobs, helping the practitioner to express and deal with the feelings content of their work
  - keeping an oversight of personal and professional boundaries to ensure that the practitioner can use him- or herself in the work but without personal needs or attitudes impinging adversely on the way the work is handled
  - talking through what to do if personal considerations look like getting in the way of doing a good job
  - enabling the supervisor to ensure that organisational policies on staff care, including worker safety, are operating effectively and that the employer's duty of care towards staff is being observed.

If this looks like a tall order, it will serve to underline why our profession has always placed such importance on supervision, and why outside observers, for example in official inquiries and inspections, have also regarded it as crucial and called for improvements to be made.

At the practical level, nothing on the above list is achievable unless supervision sessions:

● can be relied on to happen regularly
● take place in uninterrupted privacy
● offer enough time to talk (typically around 60–90 minutes)
● occur at prearranged times so that both parties can be adequately prepared and can contribute to the agenda
● are based on mutual respect between supervisor and supervisee.

Interpersonal considerations are equally vital. A mutually trusting supervisory relationship will combine clear boundaries of responsibility and accountability with the opportunity openly to air practical concerns, ethical dilemmas and more personal issues (in so far as these may impinge on the work in hand). It is because there needs to be this mutual trust that power dynamics assume such importance. There are clearly dangers in supervision where members of oppressed groups are being supervised. In so far as supervision can be seen as 'one of the vehicles through which social work organisations transmit their cultures and control their workforces' (Cosis Brown, 1998, p. 79), there is ample scope for personal or organisational intolerance to creep in. Cosis Brown points out that the private nature of supervision means it has 'rarely been opened up for scrutiny and evaluation through the processes of quality assurance'. In the context of writing about gay and lesbian staff in social work, she shows how the supervisory relationship can be anything from valuing and respectful to homophobic and repressive. Maintaining personal and professional boundaries means that the staff member must be clear about his or her own issues and needs and must not impose these on the service user. At the same time, an employee who has experienced abuse or racism or homophobia at first hand can use this personal experience to understand the pressures in the lives of those who face similar kinds of social injustice and the manager needs to understand this subtle distinction.

Models and methods of supervision

Supervision can be individual or group, formal or informal, direct or indirect. A good team manager will use several of these approaches in different contexts. Figure 6.1 shows that, working clockwise, and rotating the formal/informal pointer, this gives eight possible combinations to choose from. Thus a staff team discussing a case over lunch would be an example of informal, indirect, group supervision.

Individual supervision

Individual supervision allows for the development of professional and personal practice, recognising each staff member's stage of experience and confidence and dealing with needs that cannot be met or may be threatening in some way when talked about in groups. The individual can talk about problems that may be affecting their work and can also receive acknowledgement of work well done. This method has been the norm in social work settings and was traditionally undertaken by the first line manager, although this is decreasing the case nowadays (Kearney, 1999).

Group supervision

Group supervision (see Brown and Bourne, 1996, Chapter 9) might be chosen as the only way in which everyone will get the support they need, given the time available, but a more positive rationale is

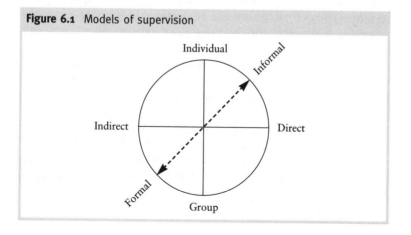

Figure 6.1 Models of supervision

that each person learns from all the others' experience and this sharing strengthens the team, making it less reliant on top-down direction. There is greater scope in a group, too, for using different methods, such as role play, case studies or sculpting. Ford and Jones (1987) add that groups reduce the impact of personality clashes or of the supervisor imposing ideas on the supervisee. In relation to staff in residential and day care, Atherton (1986) points out that the staff team in supervision might be able to rethink their approach by noticing when their own dynamics mirror issues among service users. He advises that, for this sort of learning, the group should be as small as possible, staff should be at more or less the same stage of professional development, and care should be taken to ensure that the sessions do not become management sessions or moaning arenas more appropriate to staff meetings.

Informal supervision

Informal supervision is inevitable and necessary, as one aspect of the support offered. It can be useful as an addition, either when the staff member is newly in post and needs to feel that he or she can 'pop in' for practical information or advice, or in a crisis situation when an individual needs immediate help. On occasion, too, the worker might be in the middle of an incident that holds tremendous learning potential that the supervisor witnesses – issues can be unpicked there and then, strengths pointed out and the person returned to the fray with a clearer sense of what to try next. On its own, though, informal supervision is an insufficient and inherently unreliable model. Ad hoc chats do not allow individuals time to reflect on their work or to plan the agenda beforehand, and neither do these types of discussion usually get recorded. Unfortunately, it is too easy for managers and staff who feel uncomfortable about supervision to settle for informality. But, for someone who really wants supervision, it can breed resentment because there is rarely the chance to explore all their issues. Practitioners can almost always contain anxiety and uncertainty, even if the manager's door is open, provided they know there will be a planned opportunity to discuss the issues in the near future. Managers who do not offer planned supervision, by contrast, are likely to be bombarded with unstructured queries and concerns, or alternatively excluded from vital information that they need to know.

Relying purely on informal contact is a perfunctory, dismissive and inadequate form of support, keeping workers at a distance rather than using supervision to pull people together as a team.

Formal supervision

Formal supervision, geared to developing practice to an optimum level and in which the supervisee is formally accountable to the supervisor, is distinguished by four dimensions:

1. A *structure* – needed to ensure that there is adequate preparation, regularity, a flexible agenda and time boundaries.
2. A *focus* – clear aims and objectives for the sessions, spelled out and reviewed from time to time, and even a formal learning agreement.
3. A *setting* – a context within which supervision is undertaken and which actually features as a basis for any discussions and strategies; again, the organisational context has implications for practice and thus may be at the forefront of supervisory discussions.
4. A *record-keeping system* – with a planned agenda and a note of points discussed, action to be taken, by whom and by when, and any issues that are to be referred elsewhere. Future training needs can be noted and acted upon, and both parties have a record of each supervision session, should they need to refer back to this for any reason. It may be seen as good practice to alternate between supervisor and supervisee in taking the notes.

Direct supervision

Direct supervision is fairly new to field agencies, less so in residential and daycare establishments. It is now a requirement in all the professional awards in social work that there must be direct observation of the candidate's practice in order to verify the claim that competence has been demonstrated. 'Live' supervision and sitting-in supervision are further examples of gaining direct access to an individual's practice, with scope, if appropriate, to correct any bad habits. Sometimes video/audio equipment or one-way screens might be available – especially useful for the development of micro-skills such as how to deal with hostility (Collinge et al., 1986).

Indirect supervision

Indirect supervision is normally the main approach available to most supervisors who cannot directly observe what contacts the staff member is making or what skills are employed, although in open-plan offices a great deal of information about dealings with others is evident. The supervisor has to rely on free-ranging or topic discussion methods, reading through records and possibly some experiential exercises, such as role play or simulations.

Overall, methods can be far more innovative than is frequently the case: critical incident analysis, assigned reading, role play, peer supervision and 'tag' supervision (in which supervisees supervise junior colleagues based on their own learning). An idea that could be borrowed from business is that of quality circles, where groups of between 4 and 12 staff meet once or twice a month for about an hour. They discuss how to improve the quality of their work but the immediate goal is to exchange fresh ideas, uninhibited by barriers of age, sex, status or qualification. The major benefits are that:

- ideas are used from everyone, at all levels in the organisation
- creativity and problem-solving are enhanced
- teamwork and team spirit develop
- commitment to the organisation is increased through involvement in decision-making
- understanding grows between different work groups.

Core conditions are that staff have a modicum of knowledge and skill in order to contribute meaningfully; managers have to trust people by giving them sufficient information and leeway to follow through their ideas, and it is vital that there is a coordinator.

The supervision session

A supervision session, like any interview or group meeting, has both *content* and *process* elements. The task focus (the content) is on what the worker did, why and how. At the same time, a good supervisor recognises the processes within the supervisory relationship and the session itself as occasionally needing attention.

The task discussion, for each piece of work, proceeds through the following steps:

1. *Description:* 'What happened?' to check that salient facts have been covered and understood.

2. *Clarification:* 'What did this mean?' to try to understand the situation as the supervisee perceived it.
3. *Analysis:* 'How do we make sense of it?' grounded in relevant knowledge, policy, law and practice wisdom.
4. *Implementation:* 'What are the aims in this piece of work?' and 'How can we begin moving in that direction?'
5. *Evaluation:* 'How will we know when the aims have been achieved?'

A golden rule of the supervision process is to provide both structure and space, but without inhibiting discussion. Empathic listening, establishing rapport at the outset, widening issues in the middle phase and ending the item or session with a summary, are general guidelines. With a beginning, middle and end like this, the supervisor ideally will not get caught up in an individual's real anxieties right at the end of the session when there is too little time to do anything. Assuming that there is no major problem with work performance, enabling staff to leave supervision feeling good about themselves and their work is an important aim. They should have a clear idea of any areas they could work on strengthening or gaps in knowledge that need to be filled (as well as how to do this and over what timescale) but with a general feeling of making an important contribution to achieving agreed goals. Over time, they may be able to think not just about their immediate practice but about the thought processes involved in improving it. *Reflective practice* (Schön, 1983; Eraut, 1994) refers to this ability to capture our own learning experiences so as to generalise their benefits to our broader practice. Neither theory nor technical procedures can provide ready-made answers to the complexities that social workers encounter on a daily basis (Thompson, 2002a, Chapter 24). The social worker and supervisor together can make them useful by working out what theories have to offer and where they seem to fit. After all, we clearly do need something to move us beyond the dangers of a common-sense approach to any particular situation that can be frankly wrong: 'every woman should leave violence immediately', ignoring the increased danger this can cause; 'child sexual abuse cannot possibly be widespread in the nurturing context of the family'; 'newly disabled people should adjust to living a more limited life'. Supervision is one of the key opportunities to stand back, think about practice and develop an informed analysis in place of a hunch or prejudice.

The supervisor should take away an equally clear idea of any developmental or staff care needs, as well as an overview of the person's workload, the extent to which performance standards are being met and any issues that may need taking up with another part of the organisation (for example about resource allocation or policy development). There may also be general lessons about how to make future supervision more effective.

Performance appraisal

Management methods that promote efficiency, helping workers to organise, review and evaluate their efforts, go under the general heading of 'management by objectives' (MBO). They include performance appraisal. Drucker (1954), the originator of MBO, believed that the process of planning agency-wide objectives should be one of *mutual goal-setting* between managers and staff. Unlike other planning devices, such as workload and priority systems, which frequently do not incorporate the views of those affected, the hallmark of MBO is that it tries to link each employee's goals to planned agency targets. Nonetheless, it is used by fairly large organisations in order to get everyone's commitment to top-level goal-setting, demanding that team and individual goals be consistent within this. In other words, it is still control from the top. In that performance appraisal is a part of this process, it can make staff feel defensive, particularly if badly done. On the other hand, it ensures that supervision happens and that every worker has a clear idea of what is expected of them. Also, at its best, it can be used to keep developmental and staff care needs under constant and focused review.

Top-down goals need not be arbitrary or even undemocratic. In the public sector, the agency's goals should mirror the felt and expressed needs of the community it serves. In a local authority, for example, the views of local people are meant to inform the formal plans required by government or the local democratic process. A key challenge is to find a way to combine the expectations of central government, which cannot be ignored, the views and wishes of the community, which need to be heard, and the aspirations of staff, which need to be taken into account if they are to remain committed and motivated (see Figure 6.2).

The other fear about appraisal is of having one's performance

Figure 6.2 The consultant: roles and activities

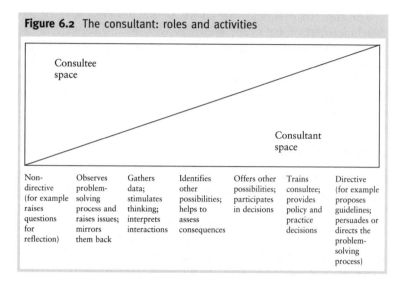

| Non-directive (for example raises questions for reflection) | Observes problem-solving process and raises issues; mirrors them back | Gathers data; stimulates thinking; interprets interactions | Identifies other possibilities; helps to assess consequences | Offers other possibilities; participates in decisions | Trains consultee; provides policy and practice decisions | Directive (for example proposes guidelines; persuades or directs the problem-solving process) |

judged. Yet there is no workplace in which managers are not forming views all the time about their staff. Traditionally, these have been unspoken and subjective, resulting in some people and not others being encouraged to apply for promotion, some being put forward for training opportunities and some being generally coached to 'get on' in the organisation. Individuals may also be put forward for pay awards in some settings. Performance appraisal formalises the process with a written record at the end. For the first time, every employee has the right to know what opinion is held about their chances of development and progression, every employee can be involved in gathering and discussing the information that underpins that judgement and every employee has the opportunity to use the normal channels of complaint if there is strong disagreement about the outcome. Those who undertake undervalued tasks, for example physical caring, can as readily be included in the appraisal scheme as those who hold professional qualifications and, if well conducted, this can improve morale in the workforce.

An effective approach to appraisal can draw on social work in more respects than the fact that it usually consists of filling in complicated forms. These include adopting the following:

- A *partnership* approach, with agreed targets, open communication and shared tasks at the outcome.
- A *systemic* approach, with agreement on what information it is relevant to input into the process, measurement from planned performance right through to outputs and outcomes and feedback to the individual so that future performance can be further improved.
- A *task-focused* approach, with agreed and prioritised goals, clear timescales (including for a follow-up meeting), shared tasks designed to reach the goals and specificity about the purpose of the evaluation, its results, and any problems as both see them.
- A *problem-solving* approach, with clear agreement as to any area of performance where competence is not demonstrated or where improvement is possible; wherever feasible tackling the immediately rectifiable ones through a personal action plan and the longer term ones through staff development, while keeping the focus clearly on strengths and weaknesses in performance, not on personal characteristics.
- An *interpersonal* approach, with use by the appraiser of active listening skills to help the staff member identify problems, reflecting back and reaching a shared understanding; also, building self-esteem through positive feedback and ending on a note of accomplishment, as well as building a positive self-image in someone who is, or is becoming, a valued member of the organisation.
- An *empowering* approach, with encouragement to employees to voice their own opinions about all elements of the process, building in self-appraisal and actively seeking comments on how the appraisal system might be improved.
- An approach based on a *written agreement,* noting agreed solutions and goals for future reference, clearly summarised.

Appraisal techniques

McKenna and Beech (1995) provide a listing of ways of conducting appraisals. The middle manager is unlikely to be given a choice of these, but the more senior manager may wish to influence the agency's appraisal system for the future. The most common mechanism is a written report, often through the completion of a standard form. This should not prove too taxing for social work managers who are used to form-filling and writing about people's strengths and weaknesses – more so than many managers in industry. MBO gains a separate listing by McKenna and Beech, as an appraisal approach in its own right.

Critical incident analysis can be used in appraisal, just as it can in selection (see Chapter 5), to gauge strengths and weaknesses from actual behaviour (which can be evidenced) rather than from more general self-report. The staff member may be asked to keep a 'critical incident log' – a running record of incidents handled well or badly (see Dessler, 1985).

Other approaches to appraisal include the use of a *development centre* to put an employee through the whole gamut of mechanisms over a period of several days, with a multi-rater, comparative evaluation being undertaken by trained assessors. This might be undertaken before deciding who to launch on an expensive training programme or a fast track for promotion.

There is no reason why *self-appraisal* cannot play a major part in several of the other systems, including MBO. It is an important part of staff development that people should learn to assess their own performance against agreed goals. The weakness in the approach includes the fact that many people in Britain tend to be modest about their own achievements and highly self-critical, with some groups more so than others – notably women and some ethnic groups (see Chapter 7). It has been found in both higher education and industry that students and workers tend to be harder on themselves than their normal assessor would be, so the appraisal needs to operate within a shared approach, with the appraiser helping the individual to recall evidence of strong points and good outcomes.

Another exciting prospect would be *upward appraisal*. Here, the subordinates appraise the manager, on the grounds that they know more about his or her detailed strengths and weaknesses over time than anyone else. Pooling views should make the process fairer. It clearly requires a major culture shift towards two-way trust and influence, however. A variation on the theme is to involve service users in performance assessment or appraisal. In practice learning, for example, there is growing interest in obtaining user feedback on student performance and there is no obvious reason why evidence of users' views could not feed into routine staff appraisals.

A process known as *360° appraisal* combines a number of these approaches, welding together the views of managers and subordi-nates with the views of other people who have worked with the individual being appraised. This requires self-confidence and a trusting and supportive structure but can offer significant rewards. In practice, any appraisal should in some way take these different perspectives into account. The formal 360° appraisal may be most effective in a staff development context, rather than as a formal annual appraisal. Yet, if service users are to be involved in appoint-ing (see previous chapter), it is a natural extension to involve them also, with others, in seeing how things work out once the appointee is in post.

A critical analysis of appraisal

As with the assessment of competences (Ixer, 1999), appraisal is only as fair as the degree to which it is possible to state what must be achieved and to which both agree on this and how to measure it. An appraisal scheme is likely to increase the power of the appraiser over groups of staff who may be operating from different sets of assumptions, and who are also more likely to be overlooked in the organisation, for example as a result of ethnicity, gender, sexuality or other social status. Indeed, in social work, the whole question of performance appraisal can be a vexed one; competence is not the same as effectiveness (as they say about medicine: 'the operation was a complete success, unfortunately the patient died'); immediate, tangible results are rare; and the notion of 'success' is saturated with uncertainties such as the intervening variables which can affect outcomes – notably, what service users and carers do themselves as opposed to what help we give them.

It is important to be clear whether the appraisal is attempting to measure behaviours, the performance of technical tasks, atti-tudes and interaction (motivation, teamwork), practice knowl-edge and skill, quality of work, volume of outputs, delivery of outcomes, organisational requirements or a combination of these. Furthermore, if an agency grasps for objectivity by using measur-ing instruments such as rating scales, checklists or critical incident logs, these are still subject to the objectivity and skill of the person making the judgements or writing the record, and the same is true of direct observation. In one interview, for example, the observer thought the practitioner should have spoken more clearly, whereas his strong local accent could have been seen as giving him an immediate advantage with service users. Even where the factors taken into account are at their most quantitative – number of cases dealt with, particular outcomes achieved, extent to which budgetary targets were observed – these are easier to measure but no easier to decide on, and not always fairer since cases vary so much. Despite the original intentions of MBO, it is rare for staff at all levels to be involved in identifying what matters most in which roles, or in agreeing ways of monitoring this.

There is a tension between using appraisal chiefly to measure individual performance and employing it to develop the workforce. These two approaches are known as 'evaluative' and 'developmental' (McKenna and Beech, 1995). In social service contexts, appraisal interviews do tend to feed into promotion procedures, whereas in some others, the emphasis may be on staff development and personal career planning, with perhaps even a choice of appraiser. Either way, it should be possible to build on strengths, so that the organisation can 'grow its own' high-fliers and future managers from among its existing staff. Overall, it can promote a *performance-oriented culture* through setting aims and providing feedback – motivating staff being one of the prime objectives of current theories of management.

Anyone who is called on to act as an appraiser, no matter what the model adopted or the techniques used, requires training and should insist upon it. It is not a bad idea for appraisees also to be offered an orientation session on the operation and purpose of their organisation's appraisal scheme. Certainly, the particular scheme to be applied needs to be well developed and properly executed, with ample time and attention given to its use in practice. The normal channels of union support, advice from a professional association, grievance procedures and even legal action are all available for use in extreme cases, where differences of view prove difficult to resolve.

Staff development

The essential combination of skill and commitment to the achievement of the objectives and service plan of social service agencies is now widely recognised. Staff development is no longer seen as a luxury, to be provided when there is some spare resource, but as a requirement. It is ironic, perhaps, that in a people-oriented service this had to be imposed from above, and was only made comprehensive because government recognised how its qualification targets for the economy as a whole would be undermined unless there was substantial investment in the social services workforce, most of whom had little training and no qualifications for the work.

The staff development plan should be an integral part of the service planning timetable and structure in any organisation, linked with a system of performance management that also takes into account the needs and interests of individuals (Horwath and Morrison, 1999). Staff development resources need to be targeted towards corporate objectives and the performance of all employees measured against operational and strategic plans. For this reason, as well as the wider ones of bringing out the best in staff and keeping them up to date, all managers need a broad understanding of their agency's staff development strategy, as well as how it relates to their specific area of responsibility and the staff they manage. They may also be asked to feed into the development of the strategy from time to time, both in detail (for example from conducting individual appraisals which reveal learning needs) and in helping to determine its overall direction (through identifying priority issues, neglected staff groups and so on).

In social services, the staff development plan is not only under the oversight of senior managers and elected members, but is also of interest to central government. A significant part of the funding for the following year is triggered by the achievement of nationally agreed training and qualification targets. The staff development strategy, including individual learning objectives, should be planned according to what the agency intends to achieve over time, that is, the *strategic direction* of the organisation. Through the identification of individual and group learning needs, staff development can meet the shortfalls in the competences and knowledge base of various grades of staff that might otherwise present obstacles to achieving organisational goals. It is essential that the aggregated findings of the staff appraisal processes feed into this planning and that it is guided by an agreed vision of how services will develop. Other factors may also be relevant, such as ensuring equal opportunities for particular groups of staff. Then, to complete the staff development feedback loop, learning is evaluated in terms of its impact in the workplace and feeds back into appraisal and future learning, not only for individuals but the organisation as a whole.

Because staff development opportunities are crucial to organisational success, managers need to evaluate the outcomes from training events. Staff will usually be expected to determine their learning aims before undertaking the training, possibly with a supervisor or mentor, and to have matched these with the learning objectives that the course or other learning opportunity specifically undertakes to deliver. Then, afterwards, staff will be expected to put their learning into practice and to comment on the extent to which the intended learning outcomes are actually demonstrated in the workplace, often through a recall day or event. In other words, learning is not undertaken for its own sake but to help people do their jobs better; and whether it works or not can be measured. A bonus of this approach is that staff learn critically to analyse their own practice (see 'reflective practice', above), to provide evidence of how it develops over time (for example in a portfolio) and identify when competence is demonstrated. They are *active participants* who take responsibility for their own learning.

Line managers have a clear role to play in this process, in that, as well as helping staff to develop skills, they are called upon to 'verify' the evidence produced. Whether done through a simple countersignature, a short written report, direct observation of practice or the production of additional evidence, it is a crucial way of proving that the claims made by the learner are genuine and, in particular, that the learning has been applied in the workplace in a manner appropriate to the practice undertaken there. Line managers may be called upon to collate information on the impact of training plans and activities to pass to strategic managers who need to see the overall picture at organisational and interorganisational level. Line managers may also need to feed back to the organisation those aspects of practice that training has revealed could be improved, for example working with vulnerable adults.

Training is not a passive process for those participating, detached from the realities of practice. Rather, it is an inescapable part not only of managing staff effectively, but also of delivering a high quality service. The Department of Health has funded the production of evaluation guidelines which outline this further (JICC, 1997).

External influence over this process of strategic planning of staff development comes in the form of government support for national frameworks of education and training. Councils with social services responsibilities are required to set targets for the numbers of their staff who will work towards these various awards. The work-based nature of much of the learning means that it can still be individualised, although government has a direct influence over content.

There is also a focus currently on management training. The main qualifications relevant to social work managers are the MBA (Master's in Business Administration) or other Master's degree or diploma in management with a public sector specialism, S/NVQs in management and the Advanced Award in Social Work (AASW). Managers constitute a further group whose needs were not well met by the old-style, in-house provision of courses mainly for professional staff, yet their role is as crucial as anyone's in meeting corporate objectives.

There has also been interest in career development for women managers (Foster and Phillipson, 1994; Foster, 1996), who are frequently isolated yet highly visible within a male-dominated management culture that prevents them from placing their particular strengths at the service of the organisation (see Chapter 7). There is some evidence that women social workers are less likely than men to have been on management courses (Murray, 1997) and that women may experience more difficulties than men in accessing training of all kinds, with problems in being selected, being freed to attend and being funded (NISW, 1998). A guide to training courses, organisations and networks for women managers is therefore of some interest (Lance and Bunch, 1998), although, having been commissioned by the now defunct Social Services Inspectorate, it is unlikely to be updated. Coyle (1989) regards specific opportunities for current women managers and women of management potential as having opened up at least a little space for women to discover their power, support each other, help others and effect change. She recognises, however, that rising through the existing hierarchy does not automatically challenge gender assumptions, let alone issues of ethnicity, class and so on.

Staff development is increasingly of concern to the whole organisation; training opportunities are not 'perks' for individual staff but one of the key ways of meeting corporate objectives. The concept of the 'learning organisation' helps to explain this (Argyris and Schön, 1978; Thompson, 2000). As noted in Chapter 3, this means not only an organisation in which learning opportunities for staff are encouraged and promoted, but also one in which the whole organisation is open to new ideas, to learning from experience and, in social work, from user feedback and interdisciplinary working. It is a question of a climate and culture in which continuous learning and self-development are valued, norms can be challenged and staff at every level are encouraged to question and explore ideas. This lies at the heart of best practice.

The effectiveness of the whole organisation, particularly in the face of rapid change, is seen as best served by *maximising people's potential*. The agency needs lively minds if it is to survive. Individual workers also need lifelong learning in order to keep up to date the portable skills that will help them to survive reorganisations or even, perhaps, to pursue serial careers with a range of employers. These trends are at odds with repressive managerialism and a passive workforce. If the role of management were seen as to inspire rather than control, having a strong management presence need not be in tension with people learning to think for themselves. Learners now need to be responsible for their own learning and to learn *how* to learn, not just *what* to learn (Thompson, 2000).

Overall, an organisation is likely to be most successful if it undertakes a training needs analysis across all staff groups to determine what organisational as well as individual training needs will best help staff to meet organisational objectives, while carrying out their roles effectively, and developing positive careers (Horwath, 1996).

Staff care

It is frequently asserted that there is low staff morale in social services. Some suggest this reflects low public esteem, arising especially from publicity about child protection cases but also poor management. It is difficult to feel relaxed about one's work when there is a 'culture of blame' within agencies, reinforced by outside comment. One of the worst aspects of a blame culture can be scapegoating – leaving staff feeling that any shortcomings in service, together with their own emotional reactions to these, are their own fault. A blame culture also generates a 'fear of failure', which blights learning, confidence and morale. An effectively operating staff development and staff care system, on the other hand, would offer the worker whose case had not turned out as hoped, first, a supported opportunity to reflect in supervision and analyse what lessons could be learned individually and by the team and the organisation and, second, the necessary personal support to cope with the personal and emotional fallout.

We cannot work with other people's pain, grief and (sometimes violent) anger without an impact on ourselves. Although we learn to deal with them professionally (focusing on the other person's needs and not our own feelings while we are with them), this should not mean that we distance ourselves from human suffering or joy so that we become cynical. In the face of chronically unmet need, social workers may negatively label service users and become rigid in applying rules. Yet 'battle fatigue' or 'working under siege' are metaphors from the workplace that suggest feeling at war with consumers in ways which managers in organisations could help to prevent. As mentioned above, part of the purpose of supervision is to help the worker to talk about the personal impact of the work. It is not healthy to the individual or their employing organisation to expect them to suppress their own emotions, avoid facing their own anxieties or deny their own stress levels. Yet this is a worrying culture in some agencies, perhaps dating from earlier times when the care of vulnerable people was seen as a vocation demanding limitless commitment. In some places, this has turned into a macho approach, in which 'giving in' to stress is seen as weakness and taking time off for illness as a needless expense to the organisation.

Stress

Thus far, we have looked at a number of ways (for example appraisal) in which organisations can protect staff from overload. This is not just about endless form-filling or lack of resources; in the human services, we often do not have the satisfaction of seeing the problems that we tackle solved and cannot rely on happy endings. With staff under constant pressure and perhaps with few intrinsic rewards, there is a risk that they will stop caring.

Much of the literature on stress talks of 'burnout' and looks for individual weakness to explain it. It explores the kinds of personalities prone to this emotional exhaustion (people without a fulfilled private life, 'workaholics', those with an unrealistic view of what can be achieved or those subject to breakdowns) and ignores the impact of organisational power structures and cultures. But, since stress-related problems rarely appear in only one person at a time, organisations need to examine in what ways their systems might erode their staff's ability to cope (Thompson et al., 1994).

Some organisations actually create a 'culture of stress' (Thompson et al., 1996) and hence put their staff at heightened risk. Workers exhibit higher anxiety and job dissatisfaction, particularly in terms of a lack of autonomy and recognition of a job well done, together with a feeling that the the job is not worthwhile because little can be done for service users within the time and resources available. The difference cannot be explained by staff characteristics or workloads. Rather, key factors appear to be line managers who have unrealistic expectations of what is possible, who give too little supervision and do not use it as an opportunity for praise, and who expect or allow work to seep into non-work time (late home visits, taking work home). They are poor at motivating and supporting their staff and helping them to organise their work, almost certainly because the managers themselves are stressed out. Since this is only happening in some organisations and not in other, comparable ones, it must be preventable through implementing a *culture change*.

Similarly, managers can be aware that there are categories of jobs in which people are more likely to be subjected to violence and so can take additional precautions for their safety. SSDs are expected by the Department of Health to provide guidance, training and support (as well as appropriate equipment) to protect the health, safety and security of users, staff and premises.

It is the risk of violence which arguably presents employers with their greatest staff care challenge. Levels of violence in SSDs are unquestionably high (Balloch et al., 1998; NISW, 1999). Developing a positive work culture to prevent and respond to the risk of violence means not waiting for incidents to happen. Staff can be routinely trained, with the emphasis on defusing potentially volatile situations and promoting their personal safety. There is now greater awareness of sensible measures that can be taken. These include physical adaptations to offices (security systems, panic buttons), workers carrying mobile phones and/or alarms when they go on visits and so on. Of course, it will not be possible to prevent all attacks. Where an incident occurs, staff must know not only how to report it, but also that something will be done about it and that they will receive support, not blame, from management in the immediate aftermath. They may also need time off work as a result of injuries or emotional trauma and longer term help in the form of specialist staff care services. There should ideally be a free, confidential and professional counselling service, independent of the employing organisation, with no leakage of information, even as to who has used the service.

There are also categories of people who face additional pressures of other kinds. Experiencing discrimination at work is enormously stressful and cannot be reduced by generalised action to lift morale (Friedman et al., 1998). It has to be tackled at source through appropriate policies and a commitment to their effective implementation. Bullying and harassment have a similar impact. Women (and a few men, for example those coping with a dependent relative at home) may be at risk of additional stress from role overload (constantly juggling demands with never any let up), role conflict (a sick child on the day a case goes to court) and role contagion (thinking about the family while at work and taking work home) (Home, 1993). Finally, anyone who is in a situation where they have to decide whether to become a whistleblower and report clear abuse or wrongdoing that is being deliberately overlooked by management cannot avoid facing enormous stress themselves (Hunt, 1998).

To sum up, the kinds of problems that can cause undue stress are:

- too much to do, especially where overload is prolonged and unremitting
- too little to do
- lack of control over the work – feeling trapped
- discrimination
- harassment
- bullying
- aggression and violence
- ill-defined responsibilities or objectives
- unrealistic expectations
- lack of supervision
- a blame culture/lack of praise
- an inflexible and unreasonable work schedule
- poor or unsafe working conditions, environment or practices
- poor working relations with colleagues
- role overload and role conflict (juggling work and home life)

● new demands with inadequate preparation (for example computerisation)
● job insecurity.

Any of these can be responded to by management, with the aim of tackling the stress-inducing factors in the working environment. Stress and workload management courses may also be helpful but it should not be regarded as solely the employee's responsibility to change.

The nature of stress

A certain amount of pressure is a natural part of life and we all experience an increase at times of exams, public appearances and so on. Our body produces more adrenalin so that we have heightened physical responses for a time. The problems arise when the pressures become excessive or unremitting, leading to stress. At first, there may be warning signs, such as an inability to shake off a cold, indicating that we might benefit from a short break. If we do not get the break or some other form of relief, things escalate, perhaps into bursts of irritability. Finally, there is a build-up into some of the following signs:

● **Physical**
  – chronic tiredness
  – insomnia
  – tension headaches and muscle pain in the upper body
  – digestive problems
  – reduced libido
  – tightness in the chest
  – heightened sensitivity to noise.
● **Emotional**
  – inability to shut off from work or see how a break can possibly be taken
  – irritability
  – constant worrying, for example about work, health
  – feelings of failure and of inability to cope, fear of the future
  – lack of concentration
  – loss of enthusiasm and sense of fun
  – anxiety and/or depression
  – mood swings
  – feeling guilty, looking for others to blame

- – feeling swamped by the job
- – loss of caring concern, cynicism.
- **Behavioural**
  - – withdrawal
  - – communication problems
  - – inability to make decisions, loss of creativity
  - – disorganisation
  - – poor timekeeping
  - – absenteeism
  - – resorting to drink or drugs
  - – overindulging in food or loss of appetite
  - – declining job performance
  - – forgetfulness
  - – accidents, for example clumsiness, car accidents with no apparent cause
  - – untidy personal appearance
  - – inactivity.

With all the above, it must be emphasised that we are talking about an otherwise unexplained change in the person's normal state or behaviour. Where someone has been a good employee and they suddenly begin to have unexplained absences, make mistakes or drop below par in their performance, it is reasonable to suppose that something is wrong, either at home or at work.

Responding to stress

If a problem is clearly job related and the problem is dealt with at an early stage, it may prevent someone experiencing a breakdown in their mental or physical health, which could cause them untold distress and be costly for the organisation. In other words, it is better to deal with the cause rather than the symptoms. There may be solutions such as an internal transfer, a change of responsibilities – perhaps including a new challenge – a holiday or period of unpaid leave to travel overseas or a move to part-time working, or there may be sources of support which can be tapped, either inside or outside the organisation.

It is now clear that the onus is on the employer, where it is already known that a stressful job has been having an adverse effect on someone, to take action to reduce the risk to their future health and safety. In a well publicised, landmark case,

Walker v. *Northumberland County Council* (1994), John Walker, a social work manager, was supported by his trade union in making a successful personal injuries claim against his employer. This was for breach of the common law duty of care, in that the organisation had failed to take reasonable steps to avoid exposing him to a health-endangering workload, after it was already clear that his mental health was suffering and despite his repeated requests for extra staff and more administrative support. This moves us well beyond the realm of personal coping with pressures into organisational measures, such as workload management (see below), clarity of priorities and procedures, adequacy of supervision, availability of resources, staff care in the face of violence and trauma, and the overall culture of listening to staff concerns and valuing their contribution. This stems from a recognition that work-based stress cannot be understood outside the working context (Pottage and Evans, 1992). Other public sector cases have raised further issues that employers may reasonably be expected to tackle, such as carrying an unreasonable workload, lacking the level of qualification and training needed to do an effective job, and suffering bullying and intimidation in the workplace (Schwehr, 1999). All these require an organisation-wide culture that sets clear expectations and supports staff in their work. At the same time, there have been other court judgements that have limited the employer's liability, notably where published procedures have not been followed. Individuals are thus seen as having some measure of personal responsibility for managing their own pressures and seeking help when needed.

Some specific methods of mitigating the stress of working in distressing and frustrating jobs include the points listed below:

1. training staff, both experienced and newcomers, in preventive techniques such as stress management and time management (see below)
2. rotating tasks and providing clear guidelines by which team members may negotiate 'time out' (that is, work which is less demanding than constant service user contact)
3. introducing flexitime to give staff control over the pattern of their working day and help them balance work, family and other outside demands

4. streamlining paperwork and computerised recording systems so that they help the work get done rather than feeling like additional obstacles
5. assisting teams to become cohesive and consistent in responding to service users, without losing compassion
6. helping staff to identify their coping styles (for example warning 'sprinters' that 'long-distance runners' fare better)
7. orienting workers' families to the job's inherent frustrations, rewards and importance
8. passing around tips for survival to one another
9. promoting physical fitness by lunch and after-hours exercise, perhaps either arranged or publicised in the workplace
10. encouraging employees to join networks outside the office
11. working on personal career plans or new projects for those who feel 'stuck' in their job
12. improving salary levels and promotion prospects, including for older workers, women and black staff
13. engaging in participatory management so that staff feel part of the overall enterprise (see Chapter 3)
14. making it clear that intimidatory behaviour will not be tolerated through a published code or codes on harassment and bullying
15. ensuring that the overall management style is not a bullying one but one in which individual and team contributions are respected and valued
16. having grievance and harassment procedures in place for staff who feel they have been unfairly treated or discriminated against
17. offering a staff care or 'employee assistance' programme (see below).

Staff care begins with a workplace culture in which staff can voice their worries and be listened to, including in regular and effective supervision, so that concerns can be addressed. A line manager can tactfully ask an individual whether there is something particular on their mind; there may be an obvious explanation for them looking unwell or stressed out, such as family illness, or they may say that the job is getting them down. It is always worth advising a medical checkup; illnesses such as chronic fatigue syndrome (or post-viral fatigue syndrome, formerly known as ME) (Shepherd,

1997), anaemia or an underactive thyroid can produce extreme lethargy.

Antidotes to occupational stress begin at the interpersonal level. Managers have to be prepared to listen and show that they care about their staff, making reasonable allowances if, for example, someone's health is temporarily below par or they are preoccupied by a bereavement. Equally, compliments on work well done are essential; managers sometimes behave as if workers were disposable. Feedback should not be reserved for times when something has gone wrong. Overall, it would seem self-evident that cared-for staff are more likely to care for the users they serve.

Clearly, though, managers must draw boundaries around their role in relation to staff and not see themselves as counsellors (a temptation when you are social work trained). A test as to whether to 'say something' to an employee who appears to be having problems would be, most importantly, whether or not the problem appears to have been caused or exacerbated by the working environment, or to be having an impact on the work of this individual or others. Other factors to consider would include whether the person concerned has sought your help, and whether or not they are already accessing appropriate systems of help and support outside. To take a tricky example, but one that satisfies the test of having an impact on the work of others, where someone's body odour is causing others to stay out of their way, a 'quiet word' is certainly called for. An example of being asked for help could be where one worker tells you that a colleague is constantly offloading work onto them; here, it would seem expedient to try and resolve these unhelpful relationships, perhaps through a team meeting on workloads and roles or a team-building exercise. Where the situation clearly lies outside the office – if someone appears to be drinking rather heavily, say, but is already getting help and their work record is improving – this might be one to monitor from a distance, unless the timekeeping or standard of work starts to slip again. A balance always needs to be struck between ducking out of intervening.

Another layer of boundaries between manager and staff comes into play where the employee needs to seek personal advice. A confidential employee assistance programme (EAP) can play an invaluable role. People need to know that the scheme can safely be approached for personal support and counselling and that it will not affect their chances of promotion or others' confidence in them as a good worker. The services offered may include short-term counselling and staff support groups.

In addition to managers looking out for signs of stress in individual staff (and in themselves), and offering individual support schemes outside, comprehensive management information can be gathered that may indicate that the organisation as a whole has a problem. A marked increase in any of the following would be indicative of something being wrong: sick leave, accidents, turnover, use of grievance and harassment procedures, complaints by service users, poor results in audits and reviews, evidence of poor teamwork, new ideas not getting off the ground, objectives and targets not being met, and a generally worrying picture emerging from appraisals and staff development evaluations. The response may need to be a complete culture change in the organisation, with the focus on valuing, developing and caring for the workforce, as well as on organising work sensibly, without taking away the rewards of personal autonomy in the exercise of skill and judgement.

Worryingly, there are some signs of organisations using their management information to become more punitive towards individuals rather than more aware of their own responsibilities. Throughout the 1990s, for example, there was growing concern about levels of sick leave but the use of the word 'absenteeism' to refer to this appears to place the blame on individuals who may, in fact, be affected by stress or unsafe or inefficient working practices (Daly, 1998). Some of the sickness monitoring procedures are experienced by staff as a first warning in a potential move towards disciplinary action, rather than as a way of finding out about underlying problems. Referees are asked to give information about employees' past sickness records, so that a move to a new job to escape unreasonable stress may also become more difficult. It is possible to combine rigorous sickness monitoring, instead, with health promotion, good staff care and an awareness of the relevance of team and workplace culture (Daly, 1998).

Workload management

Everyone manages their own work to some extent by using their diary to plan commitments and making constant decisions about when and how to perform tasks. More formal workload management, however, involves a systematic weighting of cases or other pieces of work, allocation of these up to an agreed limit for each worker and monitoring progress. It naturally involves more work for the frontline manager, including being involved in prioritising work, allocating it and balancing workloads. As with so much in contemporary social work, this brings home the lesson that employee time is a resource under pressure that has to be rationed, just as much as places in residential care and cash budgets.

Over and above the handling of the routine workload, there need to be procedures in place to cope with emergency and other unplanned demands, ebbs and flows in the work coming through and the whole question of unallocated cases, when there are simply too many users needing services from too few staff.

Workload management has links with supervision, because that is where the progress of work is tracked, and with staff appraisal. Employees need a good fit between the work they are doing and their own skills and abilities, with staff development providing opportunities to grow into new areas of work and staff care offering appropriate support, such as a temporary lightening of the load, for example. The auditing and management of workloads also relates to the collection of statistical data by the organisation and, indeed, to all aspects of strategic and operational management, in that it regulates the point at which these are translated into a service to the public.

In a profession where levels of risk and violence are high, any measures that enable team members and managers to moderate the pressures placed upon them, and to manage these within a system owned and agreed by the whole organisation, must be all to the good. On the downside, they may involve saying 'no' more often to service users and leaving some categories of work to stockpile. But at least we live in an era where audits of community need and the publishing of criteria, targets and achievements place this balancing act in the public arena and, in the local authority context, submit it to political judgement. This implies greater equity both for staff and service users and should mean that the practitioner is not left to work harder and harder to keep up with impossible demands. Having said this, few agencies have developed a workload management framework that has been sustainable and capable of consistent implementation across more than one team.

Grievance procedures

Where an individual employee does feel that they have been unfairly treated, in respect of workload or any other matter, they may wish to register a grievance. This is an action internal to the organisation, as opposed to using the courts or an employment tribunal to seek justice.

As with disciplinary procedures, any manager who is involved in the build-up to what might become a grievance would generally do well to see first whether the issue can be resolved informally. This will give the staff member a prompter response and be more likely to lead to the graceful apology or localised change that the employee really wants. At this stage, it is important for the manager to know the limits of their own flexibility to act since there may be things they can do to rectify the situation swiftly and without fuss (Pettinger, 1997).

It is equally important, though, not to leave the staff member feeling that their issue was not taken seriously and for the organisation not to leave unresolved a matter which might have wider implications. Once into a grievance, there will be both internal procedures to guide the manager and legally recognised standards against which these will have been prepared, as well as advice from other quarters on personnel and legal implications. Managers can do a great deal to create a climate in which misunderstandings can be talked through and concerns considered promptly and fairly without being 'allowed to fester and rankle' (Pettinger, 1997, p. 343).

Self-help support and self-directed learning

In addition to joining a trade union – thus benefiting from a system of support, independent of the workplace, which plays an important part in ensuring more humane and enlightened treatment of workers – and a professional organisation, staff can take steps of their own to protect their own well-being, assess their own abilities and potential, and develop their own learning and hence career opportunities. Chief among these are the establishment of informal support groups or more formalised employee network groups to supplement staff care, and self-directed learning mechanisms, such as courses taken in the evening, to supplement staff development.

Support groups and employee network groups

In the UK context, groups of this kind in the workplace typically combine support, opportunities for personal and professional development, empowerment and the development of a strengths-based approach. A support group open to those who define themselves as black, for example, will operate from black perspectives, thus basing practice on knowledge that derives from the experiences of black people, as articulated by them, and placing understanding within the context of the historical subjugation of black people and continuing racism. This relocates black people from the periphery of provision to the mainstream, and works for racial justice and equality in staffing and service delivery. A group which operates within such a philosophy provides an opportunity for black workers to feel more powerful within their own support networks, to develop a collective black identity, to critique and monitor white-dominated approaches to practice while developing alternatives, and to identify and challenge overt and covert racism within the organisation (Stubbs, 1985; Dominelli, 1997).

Some groups have to think about how inclusive they want to be. A combined group for gay men and lesbians, for example, might not be an entirely comfortable place for those lesbians who prefer an all-women environment, and the group also has to be clear that bisexual and transgendered men and women will be welcome. Similarly, a black support group will be faced with decisions about those who are of mixed heritage and those who are 'politically black', that is, who face discrimination because of their ethnic or national origin or religion, but not on account of skin colour (for example Middle Eastern or Irish people).

In addition, support group members may need to challenge one another to recognise the interactions between the various forms of oppression. Women's groups, for example, need to ensure that their agendas are not set only by young, middle-class, white, heterosexual, able-bodied women but that diversity and difference are acknowledged and celebrated in an inclusive membership and debate. Provided this inclusivity can be achieved, members of the group may find it an intense relief to relate to others in a single-sex environment where they do not have to compete with men to be heard or have their views valued. Topics they may feel freer to discuss might include women's life and career choices, life cycle issues, sexual harassment and sexual violence in the workplace, appropriate service delivery to women users and carers and assertiveness for women professionals and managers. Women returning after a career break, those who work from the isolation of home or in an intensely male-dominated environment and those who have had to take up a harassment or sexual discrimination case may be among those who most appreciate the support. Male managers have a particular responsibility not to belittle or mock women's groups, white managers not to undermine black groups and so on. Their thriving is to the benefit of the whole organisation. Women's groups have proved to be a particularly useful form of support among workers whose feminist perspective is at variance with the dominant stance of their agency (Dominelli and McLeod, 1989).

The value of support groups is in helping staff members to feel less isolated and vulnerable. They facilitate personal and professional learning about ethnicity, gender and sexual orientation and provide opportunities to explore their personal significance, so that in the workplace, workers will be confident and secure in their identities and will, in turn, be more effective. Support groups provide an opportunity for people to relax as themselves without having to be on guard against hurts or misunderstandings, to talk in a rapid shorthand based on shared understanding and get to the heart of issues that others often try to block in mixed forums. These encompass the additional pressures faced, for example, by black staff who are expected to be culturally (and often literally) bilingual, experience high-profile visibility, are expected to be 'race experts' while being overlooked and bypassed, and face racial harassment, racist comments from service users who sometimes refuse their intervention, and the risk of racial attack.

A lesbian and/or gay support group may need a level of confidentiality and privacy not requested by other groups (although there can be a 'backlash' against membership of any group), since it cannot be assumed that all those who would potentially benefit from support are 'out' in the work setting or would even want to be. The group should nevertheless be well publicised and respectfully spoken about in the organisation in order to convey that the low visibility of its meetings (perhaps out of work time and not on work premises) do not make it less important than other groups that meet more openly. In social work education, it is quite common to publicise a gay, lesbian, bisexual and trans student support group to all students, without waiting to be asked and certainly without expecting to know who attends it (Logan et al., 1996). Employment settings could usefully follow suit.

In the USA, 'employee network groups' take a strengths-based approach, pool the resources of their members for mutual support, are under the control of the members, not management, and are formally recognised by the employer, with office holders and rules. Some UK support groups do operate in this way, for example some black workers' groups negotiate with management over issues raised by the membership. Dominelli and McLeod (1989) also mention women's groups as a channel for commenting on agency policies. This is not just self-help, then, but an attempt at organisational change. Women's groups, black workers' groups and gay and lesbian groups may also want to look beyond the organisation to campaign for legal changes or in support of individuals (benefits for lone mothers, deportation cases, civil partnerships).

By way of a critique of support groups, there are one or two points to mention. First, since potential members are free to choose whether or not to attend, there may be a backlash against those who do. For example, men often do not like women having a space to meet that they are not allowed to enter. Members of groups may be seen as troublemakers. Second, groups may help people to cope with their present job, rather than helping them to advance. Social interaction at work cannot be separated out from the power dynamic. Thus, when members of minority groups seek the mutual support of interacting with one another informally, they are less likely to be meeting with others in powerful positions and remain prone to miss out on the informal communication that can help majority group members to learn the score about organisational politics and advancement opportunities. Perhaps the ideal is to have support groups running alongside many other opportunities for personal support and professional development. Friedman et al. (1998) suggest that belonging to a black network group can make people feel more optimistic about their career, by making them better able to use mentoring and less uncomfortable with a white mentor.

Special interest groups

One particular role for a special interest group might be for white people who want to recognise and challenge racism, straight staff who seek to confront their own and the organisation's heterosexism or men who aim to take responsibility for tackling sexism. Such a group can consider what actions they can take to raise their own awareness and effect positive organisational change. As with support groups, difference and diversity need to be recognised. A men's group, for example, may include black and white, gay and straight, older and younger, disabled and able-bodied men, and members from various social class backgrounds. Social injustices across all these divisions need to be acknowledged, so that no one feels shut out of the group by difference, while not allowing members to escape looking at their own sexism. The oppressed role can become a hiding place, sparing oneself from looking at one's own potential oppressiveness. Such a group may benefit from facilitation to prevent collusion developing.

Learning sets

Learning sets are like a seminar group discussing work-based issues. They have been developed for social work at the former NISW and, although there are various models available, tend to share the following characteristics: discussion of work issues, with time slots for each member; aiming for practical outcomes; a facilitative environment; external facilitation; and member-owned agendas (Darvill, 1998a). Although there is no external training input, outside expertise can be introduced in the form of written material that individuals have found useful or the facilitator may suggest.

As well as offering all the obvious benefits of mutual support and shared problem-solving, learning sets can help to foster a climate of high service standards and good management and a feeling of shared responsibility. They can be run with new, middle or experienced managers, or for those in more specialist posts in the hierarchy, but it is probably best to keep each of these separate, so that agendas are sufficiently held in common and stages of learning are similar.

Self-selected learning opportunities

As noted above, staff development opportunities in social work increasingly serve organisational priorities. There has been a shift from 'education' to 'training' (Thompson, 2000). At the same time, there has never been so much choice of part-time degree and lower level programmes available in every higher education institution and further education college in the country, many of which can be pursued in the evenings, alongside a full-time job.

In that all learning influences who we are and hence the way we do our jobs, there is no subject which will not make the social worker see the world in a fresh way and virtually none which does not have some indirect relevance, whether it be modern languages improving communication skills, philosophy giving new clarity to ethical dilemmas or sociology showing how the fabric of social life has developed over time. Learning how to learn is also important, as we saw in relation to reflective practice.

Consultancy and mentoring

Consultation can be defined as an occasional event directed towards solving a particular set of problems or promoting a particular approach to practice without involving managerial power relationships. Mentoring is typically offered to an individual and takes place over a period of time, sometimes with a particular aim in view, such as the achievement of a professional award, but sometimes directed at more general career advancement. Bhatti-Sinclair (1996, p. 9) defines the mentoring role as being to 'provide a listening, counselling and empowering role'; there can also be educational and developmental aspects. She sees the consultant as having a more active validating and advocacy role, although this is not the only possibility. Thus, both consultancy and mentoring are separate from staff supervision and line management. Often, consultation is requested by the person who receives it. Where it is 'prescribed' by management to tackle difficulties, it is unlikely to be as fruitful, but there are also some enlightened managers who perceive instances where it could be useful and negotiate this with their team.

Another use of consultation is when a supervisor cannot meet all an individual's support or developmental needs. Where a black specialist worker is supervised by a white line manager, for example, there could be issues that consultancy could explore which would simply not feel safe to raise first in supervision but which can then be taken up as appropriate.

The knowledge and skills of consultants are typically somewhat specialised and it may be hard for a manager to judge the quality of what they will offer. Nowadays, there are any number of free-lance consultants available. It is sensible to take organisational help in selection and in drawing up a contract (see Kara and Muir, 2003).

Stress management

Although the earlier section on staff care quite rightly put the emphasis on managers and on organisational culture in general as being the key elements in preventing stress (and nothing in what follows should be taken to suggest that experiencing stress is a result of individual weakness), there are ways in which people can care for themselves and manage their own pressures more effec-tively. We cannot prevent social work from being inherently one of the most demanding of jobs. Dealing with human problems and unpredictability is part of what makes it rewarding. But recognis-ing the potential for stress and learning to read, and react to, the signs of its effects on oneself (constant minor illnesses, mistakes, irritability, problems with sleeping) are sensible precautions in handling the demands before they build up into illness or burnout. Thompson (2002a) suggests the following personal effectiveness tips:

- know yourself
- set objectives
- change your attitude
- be assertive
- keep control
- set boundaries
- learn time management
- use support
- avoid unhelpful coping methods
- be kind to yourself.

Stress in a workplace also feeds on itself, as we saw above, so a team or group of colleagues might usefully decide together to implement stress reduction techniques. These can be as simple as going to a lunchtime aerobics class once a week, stopping for proper coffee breaks, putting workload management on the staff meeting agenda or arranging a talk on effective time management.

Time management

Since social work is labour-intensive, one of its most valuable resources is *time*. Many managers confess to having difficulty with time management. Here again, there are some pointers which can help, including:

- Take time before a meeting or a telephone call to think what you want from it and keep this in mind throughout.
- Keep a note of everything you need to ask key people, so that you can cover them all in one meeting or email contact.
- Have these notes to hand in case they should happen to ring you.
- Look ahead through your diary from time to time so that you can organise your time most effectively, for example organising two meetings consecutively that involve a journey in the same direction, grouping activities to release useful slots of time.
- Have meetings at your office rather than always travelling to someone else's.
- Write up notes, make a first draft of documents (or jot down the headings) while the material is fresh in your memory; this is much quicker than trying to remember it later.
- Follow up immediately on any promises made.
- Compartmentalise certain functions, for example set aside slots for recording or receiving return phone calls.
- Never have any 'dead time'; make longer journeys by train and use them for concentrated reading, use driving time to think through complex problems, recognise that time spent chatting over the kettle is valuable interaction with team members.
- Shut your door when you want to work undisturbed, but ensure that staff know when you will be available.
- Never feel guilty about working at home: you can get through mountains of work and do it carefully and well.
- Set aside time for planning and 'visioning'.
- Think in annual and other periodic cycles, not task by task (you should always know what regular work is coming up and when).
- Allocate time for administrative tasks in your diary.
- Wherever possible, only have a document in your hands once; either deal with it, file it, bin it or pass it on.
- Where the last point is not possible, group paperwork into types of task and allocate time for each, with a deadline.

● With a longer term project, always try to have one concrete step moving forward (for example doing the groundwork for the next meeting, making relevant phone calls) and work out a way for your attention to be triggered if one of these steps grinds to a halt (for example if someone fails to get back to you).

There may not be many 'breathing spaces' in the day, and yet most of us would admit to using our time unproductively at times. Others can control our time if we allow them constantly to interrupt us or draw us into what are properly their own concerns, while putting off decisions can result in crises that take longer to sort out. Other common failings are concentrating on less important jobs, never knowing when tasks should be delegated to others, and habitually overcramming our diaries so that we have no time to chat or think. It is worth re-emphasising that the commonest causes of poor time management are doing other people's work and failing to prioritise tasks.

Conclusion

This chapter has shown the range of ways in which social work organisations can foster their greatest asset, their staff, through maximising their potential, harnessing their efforts to the wider objectives of the organisation and observing the duty of care towards them. Without suggesting that any of these responsibilities be abdicated, it has also suggested some ideas through which staff can promote their own learning and well-being.

Much of the chapter has considered the workforce as if it were a homogeneous whole. Chapter 7 will explore difference and diversity in the workplace, as well as some more radical ways of celebrating a strengths-based approach to management.

7 | Managing diversity

With over 80 per cent of the social services workforce made up of women (Balloch et al., 1995), disability legislation catching up with sex and race discrimination and recent major strides in recruiting black students and staff, not to mention all the attention focused on anti-oppressive practice, we might like to think of social work organisations as being well ahead in terms of equality and diversity. A closer look, however, reveals that, despite advances, there is still a long way to go.

Anti-discrimination legislation

Legislation provides the foundation for equal opportunities in relation to access to jobs, promotion and fair rates of pay. The monitoring undertaken by the Equal Opportunities Commission (EOC) and the Commission for Racial Equality (CRE) reveals in their annual reports that the position of female and black and minority ethnic workers has not improved as much over the lifetimes of these organisations as we might have expected. Women in management and administration still earn less than men while, in social services, there is research evidence that women continue to be disadvantaged in the workplace relative to men, particularly when they have dependants (reported in Thompson, 2002b). In a similarly dispiriting vein, by 1996, the CRE could report fewer than 2600 people having had complaints of racial discrimination supported by industrial tribunals or courts (CRE, 1996), in a labour market in which black and Asian people remained twice as likely to be unemployed as white people (CRE, 1997).

A single Commission for Equality and Human Rights will in future cover not only the three existing areas of gender, 'race' and disability – subsuming the three existing commissions, the EOC, CRE and the Disability Rights Commission (DRC) – but also three new areas of discrimination in which the EU is requiring the UK government to provide protection: age, religion and sexuality. It will be in a better position to monitor progress across the board and to deal with issues that overlap, provided that some voices do not come to dominate over others.

There is a major conceptual challenge involved in moving to a new, more overarching way of conceptualising equality. Under earlier legislation, a number of shortcomings were apparent. In particular, the legal brief has been reactive and narrow, dependent on proof and interpretation, so that employment tribunals have too often found it difficult to establish that discrimination has actually occurred.

The Acts have operated on the basis of 'individual grievance', meaning that one named individual must bring a complaint of differential, disadvantageous treatment, even where a whole category of workers is affected. Without the backing of the EOC, CRE or DRC, this was too daunting for many people to contemplate or too financially risky, given, for example, that costs can be awarded against the applicant. Even with support, it is not a pleasant prospect to be cross-examined in a tribunal and can be both distressing and embarrassing, so the majority of aggrieved individuals simply never took action. The hope, now, is that it will be more effective to place the onus on the employer or service provider to prove that adequate steps had been taken to promote equality through a race equality, disability equality or sex equality scheme. A move towards this has occurred, for example, under the Sex Discrimination Regulations 2001, whereby the employer will have to prove that they have not discriminated, once a prima facie case of discrimination has been shown. This should make it easier for applicants to win sex discrimination and equal pay claims or have them settled out of court.

Although indirect discrimination is also unlawful (that is, unjustifiably applying a condition which adversely affects one particular group) proving that it has occurred is yet more difficult. For instance, there are often hidden and not so hidden agendas when candidates are interviewed for jobs. Although the Sex Discrimination Acts invalidate questions about child care arrangements, it is hard for a woman to refuse to answer a question about this if she is really keen to get the job, although she is within her rights to do so. And, while equal opportunities interviewing has at least been thought about (see Chapter 5), psychometric and other tests may remain unintentionally ethnocentric in either their content or process of operation. Because the tests are standardised around white test results, black people may find themselves valued only in as far as they conform to white norms and fewer may be appointed to posts as a result (Skellington with Morris, 1992). Similarly, GSCC regulations on health and fitness to practise as criteria for social work registration, if rigidly imposed, could rule out many people with physical disabilities or histories of mental health problems who would, by any objective measure, be perfectly well able to work effectively.

If a case is taken, even if successful, the complainant may subsequently be undermined by colleagues or managers, being made to feel incompetent and patronised, and it is particularly hard to document attitudes and behaviour that pervade the very culture of the workplace or to take action when many people are involved. Research in Northern Ireland (EOC for Northern Ireland, 1998) revealed that, although most were pleased overall that they had made an enquiry or complaint, almost a third of the 859 respondents had experienced a deterioration afterwards in relationships with colleagues, one in three had suffered some form of victimisation, and almost a fifth had gone on to a period of unemployment following their complaint. A test case in England does mean, however, that victimisation after challenging a decision or action based on racism or sexism is itself covered by the discrimination legislation (*Community Care,* 30 September–6 October 1999, p. 17). This is vitally important because many members of socially oppressed groups have probably experienced harassment in the workplace and taken no action, not through weakness but after a conscious calculation that either nothing will be done anyway or that they are likely to suffer worse repercussions than their harasser (Coleman, 1991).

There is a crucial difference between equal opportunities and anti-oppressive thinking. The former works from a position of treating individuals equally (in this case, in the labour market), which usually means, for example, treating women more like men, whereas opposing oppression means tackling global injustice against women by a more fundamental rethinking of gender power dynamics. The announcement by the EOC in 1996 that, for the first time in its history, its annual workload included more individual complaints from men than women starkly reveals the weakness of an individualistic approach. Equity-based European thinking has been even further wide of the mark, with encouragement to men to move into traditionally female-dominated areas of employment, such as day and residential care of young children (Gensen, 1996), as part of evening up the numbers across all types of jobs without heed for the potential dangers (Pringle, 1992/3). The entrenched issues of violence, abuse and the exploitation of power are simply not on this kind of equal rights agenda.

In recognition of the limitations of the narrow, individualistic, legislative approach, there has more recently been a move towards 'mainstreaming' equality through overarching approaches and this is now EU and UK governmental policy. It means that every policy discussion and decision taken should be considered for its discriminatory implications, to ensure that it will not result in any group being treated adversely. The onus moves to the employer or the service provider to consider how all relevant people will be affected, instead of identifying and raising ways in which they may be being discriminated against. Recent legislation, such as the Race Relations Amendment Act 2000 in England and Wales and section 75 of the Northern Ireland Act 1998 (covering religious belief, political opinion, ethnic group, age, marital status, sexual orientation, gender, disability and dependency), requires public authorities to produce equality schemes. There is an equivalent duty to promote equality of opportunity placed on the Welsh Assembly. This is a proactive, rather than an individualised and reactive approach – a real advance on the past. The same approach can be taken wider than the public sector, for example, requiring all employers to take preventive measures, set out within their equality plan, to prevent sexual harassment in the workplace, or if the voluntary sector responds to a call from the CRE to help it police the response of public bodies to their new legislative responsibilities on racial equality. This approach is spreading to other forms of discrimination as disability and gender equality schemes will also be required. Once baseline policies are in place, 'gender, ethnic or disability auditing' can provide a way of employers themselves looking for hidden discrimination within the functioning of their organisations and incorporating issues of social justice into strategic planning.

Equal opportunities policies

Staffing

Every organisation should have an equality policy and can use it as a challenge to think beyond the confines of anti-discrimination legislation and towards implementing more widespread and pro-active measures to assist oppressed groups in the workplace.

It is important to recognise that legislation makes positive discrimination as unlawful as negative discrimination and that there is a limitation of reasonableness on the adaptations that employers have to make to avoid treating disabled applicants less favourably. To offer someone a job simply because they are female, black or disabled is not permissible, unless the post is exempt from the provisions of the relevant Act, for example because it is based in a women's refuge, in which case the claim for exemption should be stated in the advert. To do so would give any man, white or non-disabled applicant who felt they had been passed over immediate grounds to claim unfair treatment. Also women, black and disabled staff themselves may be among those who feel most strongly that no favours should be given to particular candidates; they should fit the criteria and not have to feel less 'worthy' of a place or open to accusations or unspoken comments from others that they got on through patronage. Affirmative action quotas in the USA have come in for these kinds of criticisms because it is felt that not all black students have got into university on equal merit. Against a history in the USA of slavery and segregation, and with a different legislative framework, it is important not to assume direct comparisons with the UK nor to underestimate what has been achieved by this policy. Bowen and Bok (1998) argue that black students admitted to places have achieved better outcomes than the excluded white students would have done (the latter being the least able of their cohort) and that they constitute vital 'social capital' for their nation. Nevertheless, the ferocity of some of the debates in the USA might give us pause for thought.

Positive action, on the other hand, is seen as an imaginative way forward in the UK and does not involve altering the rules in the same way as affirmative action (which here we call 'positive discrimination'). Crucially, positive action does not violate the principle of employment and promotion on merit, because it implies reaching out rather than giving special treatment to the target population once reached. Monitoring the workforce against the national and local populations gives a measure of which groups are underrepresented in employment terms. Targets (but not quotas) may then be set as to the percentage of women, disabled people and members of ethnic minority communities who ought by rights to be in the workplace, preferably with action timescales set for change. It is important to break down both the action and the intended targets by grades of staff, since there may be, for example, a good number of black women in the workforce but largely confined to the lowest paid, low-status positions.

The issue of outreach in recruitment was touched on in Chapter 5. The social work press, for example, often carries advertisements saying that the employer would particularly welcome applications from certain underrepresented groups, but efforts can go beyond this into publicising posts and raising the organisation's profile and credibility in, for example, local black communities or disabled people's organisations. Adaptations to the workplace have to be made in advance of disabled people applying and finding themselves disadvantaged by being unable to work in the organisation. This includes major work to make buildings more accessible. Staff development was tackled in Chapter 6 and, again, there is an enormous amount that can be done, such as offering women-only courses and courses for black staff, support groups for those who aspire to get into management, mentoring and consultancy schemes, and opportunities to 'act up' in posts that otherwise might seem unobtainable.

Unfortunately, it is all too easy for employers to boast that they have an equal opportunities policy and state this in job advertisements when, in reality, there may be no accompanying resources and only limited commitment to improve policy or practice.

Service delivery

Equal opportunities extend beyond staffing considerations into service delivery. It is vital to consider whether the agency currently discriminates against any particular groups of service users, either wittingly or unwittingly, in its commissioning and/or provision of services. Here again, management information can be gathered as to whether men and women, members of different ethnic groups, residents in different parts of the town or rural areas and so on all use the service in numbers commensurate with their presence in the relevant population. With the more hidden populations, it will be harder to gauge whether take-up is skewed but equally important to ensure that services are appropriately publicised and made accessible and acceptable to all. Thus, gay and lesbian service users should be directly referred to in the policy and considered in the provision of all services and the training of staff. Would every group care setting give a warm welcome to a gay or lesbian partner of a resident or centre user? Does every children and families team value lesbian and gay parenting? These are concrete questions that will make an enormous difference to the quality of life for these groups of service users.

It is important that we do not neglect our own part in the culture of our employing organisation. The personal views of a staff group may well influence the service provided. Hardman (1997), for example, conducted a survey in a local authority SSD and a postgraduate social work programme, using an attitudinal questionnaire and two case vignettes. The 75 respondents were predominantly straight white women, of whom 6 out of 10 said they had a lesbian colleague or friend and 35 per cent had knowingly worked with a lesbian service user. Although more than 1 in 5 had strong views that heterosexism is the main problem facing lesbians in society, it is extremely worrying to find that almost as many took a general view that lesbians should be referred for psychiatric help (with two strongly believing this) and 1 in 10 saying they would be afraid to be alone with a lesbian. Those in child and family social work were more likely than others to believe that lesbians should not be in charge of children, while the number of women respondents in this study who were disgusted by the idea of two women having sex together does not bode well for the profession's general ability to counsel young people who may be confused about their sexuality. Further clear evidence of the persistence of pathological attitudes has been gathered in mental health settings (McFarlane, 1998). Fortunately, there is also a growing literature on gay-affirming approaches to intervention (Burstow, 1992; Sanderson, 1993; Davies and Neal, 1996).

Overall, the need is no less acute than it ever was for us to consider how discriminatory our own practice may be and how we can go about making an active contribution to developing anti-oppressive practice in our work setting, as well as how to evaluate the success of any measures adopted for personal or organisational change. Researching the culture of an organisation, for example by conducting an 'equality audit', might be a good place to start (Parkin and Maddock, 1995).

Representativeness in the labour market

Let us now look in more detail at developments in the staffing of social work and related agencies. Flexibility has tended to lead to the creation of more temporary and part-time jobs in all sectors of employment. Workers in these less secure positions operate on the 'contractual fringe' of the labour market (Handy, 1995, p. 77). Women, as society's reserve army of labour, are likely to be disproportionately represented there. A good place to observe this is in university contract research, including in the discipline of social work.

In social services, many women have gained, in terms of the pressures of daily life, from employers' greater willingness to create permanent jobs with hours which fit in with domestic commitments, but this has not necessarily helped their promotion prospects and still has not given them as much leisure time as men (Franks, 1999). Nearly a quarter of field social workers work part time, which includes more than nine times as many women as men, but the major expansion has been up to, and especially at, team leader level (LGMB and the ADSS, 1993). Men still heavily predominate at the more senior managerial levels, where part-time working would tend to be at the very least disadvantageous and usually still unimaginable.

Despite the fact that the pioneers of social work in the USA and the UK were women – Jane Addams, Bertha Reynolds, Charlotte Towle, Mary Richmond, Eileen Younghusband – and that there were many excellent women managers in the early days, for example in the children's departments of the first two decades of the British welfare state (Carter Hood et al., 1998), more recent decades have seen a male takeover of the management of social work. In 1997, of 185 directors in England, Wales and Scotland, only 38 were women, or fractionally over 20 per cent. Scotland had a better record than England (with around a third, but still not a representative number of women) and Wales far worse (only one woman) (figures extrapolated from Foster, 1997). Women had actually been losing ground in the metropolitan boroughs and London, although gaining somewhat from a lower base in the shire counties.

Joy Foster (1997) gathered evidence that women wait until they are extremely well qualified and experienced before applying for these top jobs, target their applications where they believe they have a chance of success, and sometimes adopt a male style of presenting themselves at interview (assertive language, power dressing), which is not necessarily their characteristic style of managing. Many still report encountering discriminatory attitudes during the selection process, particularly from elected members and especially during the informal stages, such as over dinner or lunch, when there may be a feeling of not being listened to or even of having dismissive comments passed. And, since some of the obstacles that work against women in other employment sectors, such as lack of qualifications and permanent jobs, do not apply in social work, the key barriers to women's advancement clearly must boil down to these discriminatory attitudes and unequal family responsibilities. Women who do make it in management are more likely to be single or divorced and without children than their male counterparts (Balloch et al., 1995). New female entrants to the profession are no less ambitious than male (Murray, 1997), so the challenge is there for organisations to help them make it to the top.

There also remains a scandalously low number of black senior managers in social work. For some time, one strand of implementing anti-racist practice has been seen as the need to employ more black and minority ethnic workers. But, instead of opening up mainstream opportunities for career advancement, the creation of 'section 11' posts under the Local Government Act 1966, to attract government funding for work in black communities, meant that many recruits were 'locked onto career ladders with virtually no rungs on them' (Dominelli, 1997, p. 145). Jobs secured under this arrangement were often temporary and somewhat sidelined, with workers liable to be exploited at the lowest levels and often pigeonholed as the department's 'race experts'. Their career launch in such posts has not solved the entrenched problem of failing to attract and promote more black managers. Between 1998 and 2001, the number of black directors of social services doubled – all the way from one to two – out of a total of 136 in England and Wales (*Community Care,* 14–20 October, 1999, p. 11 and 4–10 October, 2001, p. 15).

A similar phenomenon has happened with disabled workers, who, where they have been thought about at all, have typically been recruited into a post such as 'social worker for the blind' (rarely 'for blind people'), if they also happen to be blind, or into a hospital setting where there is already good wheelchair access and little expectation of home visiting. Yet disability discrimination legislation now makes it quite clear that there must be no barrier to a disabled people applying for or being appointed to any post for which they are the best candidate and that it is the employer's responsibility to take reasonable steps to adapt the workplace or existing working practices to remove such obstacles (Minister for Disabled People, 1996a, 1996b). It remains to be seen whether the law will prove enforceable and whether its definitions will be more inclusive than exclusive of categories of disabled people. We still await test cases as to what constitute 'reasonable measures' to ensure that someone is not discriminated against and hence indications of what changes can reasonably be expected.

Those members of oppressed groups who do make it into the upper echelons may also encounter subversion or hostility from other staff. Black managers, for example, are likely to find that some white subordinates do not know how to relate to them as authority figures, double-checking their advice with white staff at an equivalent or even at a more junior level to the black manager, reacting with particular surprise, mistrust or anger when a black manager draws attention to a weakness in their practice and so on. The racist content in these reactions may be covered by a veneer of politeness, but it is deeply ingrained and it is undermining to black managers, who need to be assured that white colleagues alongside and above them in the hierarchy do not collude with it. The organisation needs to find ways to make it clear that it requires staff to face such attitudes in themselves and seek to change them, because they will not be condoned, in however subtle a form. Unless the organisational culture moves in this direction, it is unlikely to offer an acceptable service to black users and carers or to provide a supportive and appropriate environment for black staff. The equivalent is also true for disabled workers and women within the workplace. It is those who do not believe that new managers will do a good job who have the problem and who should be challenged if their remarks or behaviour make this apparent.

Opening up our thinking about work

So far in this chapter we have looked at ways of involving members of oppressed groups more representatively in personal social service organisations. The problem with this, if it remains the only change that is made, is that it can mean entering an agency's workforce on the terms set by those who got there first and who have already determined the agendas of assumptions, priorities and even language. This can lead to tokenism, harassment and continuing oppressive treatment. These, in turn, can mean that positive action measures do not work (because potential applicants are turned off by what they hear from others about the organisation or their first impressions of it) or that people who take up jobs there do not stay in them for long.

Oppression is built into the very structures of many organisa-tions because of the fundamental thinking on which they are based. The pure bureaucracy (see Chapter 2) is premised on the separation of the public and the private. Work becomes a place governed by rules, regulations and procedures. All that matters are technical qualifications to undertake a task and the maximisation of work-ing efficiency. This model of rationality sees women as making a less worthy contribution, for example if they take time off to look after sick children or need altered working hours to fit around child-rearing, since these matters are traditionally regarded as irrel-evant to work-based considerations. 'Gender, sexuality, reproduc-tion and emotionality are outside organizational boundaries, continually and actively consigned to that social space by ongoing organizational practices'; and, as a consequence, 'complex organi-zations play an important role . . . in defining gender and women's disadvantage for the whole of society' (Morgan, 1986, p. 259). It is equally the case that black staff, gay men and lesbians, disabled and older workers or those from different social backgrounds may well not feel that they 'fit' the prevailing culture of the workplace or the image held in the minds of those who control promotion opportu-nities. The strengths of what they have to offer in terms of life expe-rience, diversity and richness of contribution, and common understanding with whole groups of service users simply do not get onto the agenda.

But pressure on bureaucracy to change has started to come from the recognition that the achievement of equality of opportunity for staff can, in turn, lead to a better service being offered and that this will require fresh thinking. Contrast, for example, the old, 'Don't bring your family problems to work' approach with the provision by enlightened employers of a workplace nursery or crèche; this allows people to bring not the family problems but the family to work! Organisations are, after all, not peopled by automata, people invest their personalities and feelings in the workplace and, in turn, they are affected by the way they find themselves treated there. Attracting and retaining the best staff, and encouraging them to give of their best, means not cloning the next generation of managers in the image of the last. Some of the moves towards quality and excellence that we saw in Chapter 3 allow more space for these considerations than either the ideal-type bureaucracy or new managerialism is equipped to do.

A celebration of difference: the feminisation of management

A major shortcoming in a typical, liberal, equal opportunities approach can be that it denies difference, both within and between groups, by seeking to have everyone treated the same, whereas there may be more to be gained from celebrating it. A celebration of difference can lead to the discovery of a great variety of new strengths and skills that a diversity of women, black people, disabled people, older workers and others can offer to the workplace.

An interesting example is recent thinking about the 'feminisation of management'. Just as the English language, until challenged, made women invisible for much of the time (chairman, headmaster) and continues to denigrate the female when visible ('goose', 'bitch', 'mistress' all have derogatory meanings, while their male equivalents do not) (Spender, 1990), so classical management theory concerned itself with men managing men in masculine ways, while women disappeared from consideration (Hearn and Parkin, 1995, p. 19). Or, where they became inescapably visible through pregnancy and motherhood, women were devalued because childbearing and child-rearing were regarded as obstacles to the search for ultimate efficiency through the imposition of universal rules. Now, attitudes and behaviour that women more typically display are beginning to be valued in their own right.

Certainly, contemporary organisations require highly developed listening and communication skills in order to be responsive to their customers or service users (Peters, 1988). They also need empowering (Peters, 1988) and collaborative, alliance-building styles of management (Kanter, 1989) in order to cope with the ever increasing speed of change. No manager can expect to keep up with the technological revolution single-handed, for example. He, or she, will simply *have* to listen to other people, and work effectively with them, if the whole enterprise is not to suffer. This is sometimes summarised as 'emotional intelligence' (EQ) (Goleman, 1996) and it encompasses self-awareness, managing one's own emotions and relationships with others, communication skills and personal style, as well as the more traditional self-motivation. Women may also be excellent innovators because they have to challenge organisational and management orthodoxies (Maddock, 1999).

The research finding that, in single-sex conversations, women tend to take turns and develop one another's thoughts while men more typically adopt competitive posturing and try to dominate (Spender, 1990; Tannen, 1995) is beginning to be mirrored in management training courses. Single-sex tasks encourage participants to become aware of how they work together and how they might do so differently to achieve shared goals. Suddenly, women's talk is not 'gossip' but networking, not 'chat' but cooperative problem-solving. As the demands faced by organisations and the lines of communication they must maintain become more complex and less predictable, so women's ways of communicating, cooperating in teams, networking and drawing out each other's strengths rather than competing start to become ways of making organisations more effective. Thus, women's more natural management style is becoming equated with 'good management'.

Up to now, there have been only disadvantages for women in the fact that, while men's talk involves 'bantering', self-promotion and putting others down, women tend to avoid what they regard as boasting, play down their own authority and help each other to contribute. Without a shift of perception about communication styles, women can simply be overlooked or be seen as less able in relation to actual or potential leadership roles. When men and women are in meetings together, women who do speak up tend to find that men repeat their ideas as if they have just thought of them and then take the credit. (Or, worse still, men simply look bored until they get a chance to interrupt.) But, looked at in terms of the good of the organisation rather than the ambitious individual, it may be the women who are putting forward the people who deserve to be noticed and who are helping the fruitful ideas to emerge from discussion.

To avoid essentialism or biological reductionism in all this, it is important to remember, first, that we are talking about masculine and feminine styles, not about all men and all women. Not all men operate in a masculine style, nor all women in a feminine style. Second, we are dealing with how women and men have been socialised to be – men competitive, aggressive, status conscious, territorial; women more self-effacing, good listeners, better with people – not how they potentially could be. But, until the social rules are changed, it is important to remember that those who behave outside the norm may lose respect rather than gain it, with men being seen as 'wimps' and women as bossy. So the stereotype is hard to overcome, even if it is neither biologically determined nor universally adopted. Third, diversity and difference within social divisions are as marked as those between them. Thus there is nothing to say that a black woman, a lesbian or disabled woman would automatically feel any more heard or helped in a meeting by a white woman than by a white man. It is still likely to require personal and organisational efforts at greater inclusiveness and anti-oppressive working before true cooperation and shared decision-making can be achieved. But, whatever the complexities, the need to move away from harmfully 'macho' (and white supremacist) values in management is by now undeniable.

It is not difficult to extend this realisation into an understanding of some of the reasons why workplaces can be intensely uncomfortable for gay and lesbian staff members. Not only is there too often crude homophobia and heterosexism in much of the daily conversational interplay, but there is typically a maintenance of rigid gender hierarchies, which devalues women as women and rewards only those men who act out the expected sex role. There is beginning to be a literature on this. Hearn and Parkin (1995) and Wilson (2003), for example, offer a broad discussion of sexuality as it is embodied, expressed and overlooked in the workplace.

No doubt the ideal lies in taking the best from all management styles. Thus, the challenge for women – all women, including black women, lesbian women, older and younger women, disabled women and women who began life without socioeconomic advantages – is to be appropriately assertive without playing the competitive male game. And, in all of this, it will not just (or even predominantly) be women who need to change, but men too, since they currently disproportionately hold the power in organisations. Here, too, there is beginning to be theorising about the ways in which managements and masculinities reinforce one another and about how both might be transformed (Collinson and Hearn, 1996). There is also work which suggests that male practitioners should reflect carefully upon how they operate in organisations, and even whether they should absent themselves from whole areas of work, such as that directly involving sexually abused children (Pringle, 1992/3). Equally, they arguably have a special responsibility to establish groups and projects that work for change with sexually violent men, and in all settings where young men could usefully reconsider prevailing models of masculinity, for example in probation (Bensted et al., 1994; see also Mullender, 1996, Chapter 9, on the need for accountability to women in such work).

As mentioned above, it is by no means only women who enter a hostile world when they breach the environs of the manuals, flow charts and other rational management tools. Black managers may very well be seen as having 'sold out' by their own communities, on the one hand, and as overidentifying with service users if they speak too much about racism, on the other. Black managers may also be resented by white staff who feel there has been a role reversal. This can operate quite subtly, with staff circumventing the black manager's authority or regarding him or her as aggressive or arrogant when a perfectly straightforward request is made. Such attitudes undermine the confidence and competence that managers are expected to convey. This is doubly difficult for a black manager who is already highly visible in the organisation. Additional pressures may come from black colleagues, younger family members and others who look up to the black manager as a role model and for whose sake it becomes vital to succeed.

The pressure of having to appear confident in the leadership role, together with the weight of carrying all the responsibility for developing anti-racist services on one's own or always being the one to draw attention to the agency's shortcomings in this regard, plus being perhaps the only or the most senior black manager in the organisation, can become overwhelming. Added to this are being on the receiving end of open (and unspoken) racial attacks from colleagues and service users inside and outside the agency, having to sit on one's justifiable anger and resentment or else experiencing the exhaustion of having to express them politely over and over again, while all the time seeing very little if any change in the surrounding organisation. It is little wonder that some black managers resign. Thus, while the agency might have a good record in recruiting people from black and Asian communities, organisations that leave people to struggle thereafter are likely to frustrate the new manager's ability to do a good job. If, on the other hand, what is seen as threatening about the black manager is turned into a challenge to the organisation to change, all sorts of exciting possibilities may be opened up (Bond, 1996).

There has been some useful work on ways of encouraging and supporting women and black staff to get on in their organisations. Starting with women, specifically for social work, the then SSI (Nottage, 1991) researched first the scope of the problem – a preponderantly female workforce in local authority social services but only a small minority of women directors – and then the types of management development and training that women had received or would have valued (Allan et al., 1992). Ideas that emerged included:

- help with career development and planning career moves
- being well prepared for each move, including through acting up in a more senior post, so as to overcome the problem of women often not believing in themselves
- secondments, job swaps and project work as other ways of gaining relevant experience prior to promotion
- management training, including 'women into management' courses.

Equal opportunities policies in recruitment and selection were regarded as essential, while lack of child care provision and failure to value collaborative and participative styles were still seen as a problem. Staff development measures, such as mentoring, appraisal, support networks and action learning sets, were mentioned as valuable.

The problem, then, is not personal but structural (see Cockburn, 1991; Tanton, 1994). Both the SSI studies confirmed that: 'Women . . . do not lack ambition, but they often lack support and encouragement. They are more interested in doing a job to their own standards and exploring their own creative potential than conforming to (male) organisational expectations or seeking power or status'

(Nottage, 1991, pp. 25–6; see also Allan et al., 1992, p. 13). They may prefer to stay close to other women and to 'people-oriented' jobs, rather than accept the isolation, patronising attitudes and sometimes downright hostility higher up the organisation (Coyle, 1989). In the Nottage (1991) study, black women were particularly keen on mentoring and external consultancies, no doubt because their daily experiences of racism and being undermined were not well understood within mainstream line management support structures. The programme of SSI work led on to a helpful career development guide for women in social work and social care (Foster, 1996; see also Foster and Phillipson, 1994). Coyle (1989) regards women-only initiatives, such as employer-sponsored management training courses, as valuing women's contribution and helping participants to become potential agents for change, both for themselves and for other women in the organisation. She acknowledges, though, that access to such opportunities may be controlled and that they do not inherently challenge existing hierarchies of gender, ethnicity or class.

Across the public services more widely, there has also been work on the development of black managers (Office for Public Management, 1995; Andrew, 1996). Black managers emerged as much more distanced than white from their organisations' training and equal opportunity objectives, even though those surveyed were people who had already 'made it' into middle and senior management posts. Black managers felt persistently undermined and that their credibility was doubted and any failures homed in on. Having just begun to arrive in middle management in any numbers, black managers felt that they had been disproportionately affected by 'delayering' (cutting out the middle levels of management), and, more generally, the pigeonholing of black staff into equalities or race relations jobs had blocked career progression, both through sidelining and because a wider lack of commitment to change meant they had had few successes on which to stake a claim for advancement.

Once again, then, the structural issues outweigh the personal (both in problems and solutions), although it is no wonder that, in the light of all the above, lack of self-confidence and feelings of isolation within a hostile environment also take their toll for some. The barriers listed in the Office for Public Management (1995) study will require deep-seated change. They include negative stereotyping, marginalisation and tokenism, outright racist attitudes persisting in some quarters, backlash, excuses and dual standards. The commitment to change is seen as needing to come from the top, which inevitably equates with senior managers being prepared to give up some power and avoid cloning themselves when making high-level appointments. In local authority settings, as mentioned in Chapter 5, it will also involve elected members being prepared to appoint people from social groups they have not previously seen doing the jobs in question (which links into the wider questions of ensuring that we elect councillors who are representative of their local areas and then training them to carry out their duties).

Revisiting organisational structures

But sometimes people get tired of trying to fit into an alien environment and simply want to work somewhere where their values and philosophy of life represent the norm rather than 'the other'. A key aspect of the richness we can celebrate in UK social work is that organisations do exist which are run wholly by members of particular oppressed groups. These have often arisen because of the vacuum in essential services left by the large public authorities but, even so, their existence has given the opportunity for the people most directly concerned to set their own agendas and priorities, sometimes with interesting organisational results. Such projects include black voluntary agencies like projects for young black people in care or black people with HIV/AIDS, all-women organisations including Women's Aid groups and Rape Crisis Centres – sometimes run solely by minority ethnic women, as in specialist Asian refuge services, or by lesbian women, as in lesbian helplines – gay and lesbian projects offering advice and help to young people or wider populations who are coming to terms with their sexuality, older people's groups, disabled people's organisations, groups of young people in care, and locally directed projects in deprived inner-city areas running credit unions, tenants' groups and so on.

The black voluntary sector has grown in importance to the point where umbrella groups have begun to spring up to safeguard and promote its interests. The Black and Ethnic Minority Infrastructure in Scotland (BEMIS), for example, commissioned a survey of all 558 black and minority ethnic groups then identified north of the border, which revealed insecure funding that threatened their ability to plan ahead and even survive (McKay, 1999). Important work is also undertaken by the REU (formerly Race Equality Unit) which, for well over a decade now, has been drawing attention to the shortcomings of the personal social services in the mainstream (see, for example, Butt and Mirza, 1996) and championing the cause of black projects (Jones et al., 1992).

And, in the same way, there are gay and lesbian businesses and welfare organisations, the former not always credible to the mainstream, the latter serving needs that have typically been overlooked by the welfare authorities. Cosis Brown (1998) discusses the advantages for gay-run organisations in helping gay and/or lesbian service users to define their own needs and retain control of the knowledge, skills and values that are perceived as relevant in meeting them.

Naturally, the central argument has to be that overt and covert sexism, racism, disablism and homophobia in the funding and provision of services are unacceptable and must be eradicated, but this does not mean that the emergent women-only, black, disabled people's and gay and lesbian business and welfare organisations are not developing new frameworks that are innovative and exciting in their own right. Gay organisations, for example, have developed wholly new protocols on organisational principles, such as confidentiality and recording, and new patterns of service, such as buddying, in the context of AIDS projects. Similarly, it was disabled people's organisations that developed the social model of disability into concrete responses, such as schemes for integrated living, peer counselling and disability equality training.

As with the women's groups in the early 1970s, which began to establish services in response to women's priorities such as sexual (including domestic) violence, so the greater diversity of projects now, although beset by constant funding crises, reflects a more complex understanding of human need matched by more appropriate patterns of response. The challenge to the large public agencies is to listen, learn and emulate where appropriate, not to default on whole areas of service need because others are operating in that field – even where those others can attract commissioning funding from the public agencies through block service contracts – since that will leave the commissioners, together with all the other service providers, uninfluenced by change. Complexity should mean that we all learn from the best in what each of us is doing.

Conclusion

Unless deliberate attention is paid to the matters raised in this chapter, organisations are bound to take on the dominant culture of the society in which they are located. It is ironic, to say the least, that just when large social work agencies have bought into the managerialist ethos of a generation before, management theory itself has begun to open up to feminised and otherwise far more flexible ideas on personal qualities to value, ways to approach problems and so on. It could have been so much more fruitful for the nation if social workers had continued to value their interpersonal and groupwork skills throughout and had put these at the service of industry and commerce, rather than the influence having been largely in the other direction, with private sector-style managerialism pervading the public sector, while industry and commerce reinvent the wheels of listening, networking and respecting people.

But the social work profession, at the grassroots, does retain priorities of its own. Organisations or departments established specifically to deliver social work or related services may be thought to have a special responsibility to consider issues of gender, ethnicity, culture and religion, age, disability and health, class and poverty, and issues affecting gay and lesbian people, since these are now recognised as essential considerations in the delivery of social work itself at the practitioner/service user level. They should also, therefore, be seen as essential considerations to social work organisations as purchasers or providers of services and as employers. The many levels at which these considerations become relevant provide us with our challenge for change in the future, both in management thinking and in the design of organisations able to be responsive to the full range of human need and potential.

8 | Conclusion

So what of the future? Can the tremendous pace of change that has marked recent years in social work be sustained or will we enter a period of consolidation? There is certainly no sign at present of things standing still.

In the first edition of this book, Veronica Coulshed was keen to persuade social workers why they needed to understand that they worked in organisations with concerns wider than their own day-to-day practice and, hence, why management and organisational theory was relevant to them. Today, no such persuasion is needed. The mixed economy of welfare has become the norm and all social care organisations operate a more or less sophisticated performance management system. This means that not only do social workers have a clear awareness of the overall remit and resources of their own agency, but they also gain the wider perspective that is born of the influence of targets and performance measures and the complex links between purchasing and providing, and between statutory and voluntary agencies and very often through multidisciplinary working as well.

As this awareness has grown, the affinity with wider organisational theory has become more apparent. The importation into social work of management thinking – with its targets, standards, management information and talk of people as 'human resources' – has also made public sector management feel like a much closer cousin of business and commerce than might once have been the case.

But does this mean that today's social work manager has to adopt the stereotype of a macho business ethos and be ruled by it, or does a study of the management literature reveal choices in the way things are run? It has been one of the intentions of this book to demystify much of the technical language and reveal that, while psychometric testing, outcome measurement and the like may sound scientific, any student of the social sciences is well equipped to perceive the limitations as well as the advantages of an overly managerialist approach to management and to decide how far to be influenced by it. Of course, it is an advance to make clear statements to users and carers about what standards services aim to achieve and the extent to which this is managed, but people cannot be turned into simple numerical units without losing sight of much that is best about social work and the principles that have traditionally sustained it. Those human service organisations that serve people best understand effective management and ensure that its practice is grounded in the humanitarian ethics and principles that should guide management and practice alike.

Personal style and principles: time to invent anti-oppressive policy?

It comes as a welcome insight, then, and for some perhaps a surprise, to learn that there are other trends in management – that there is a choice of managerial styles to adopt, a range of visions to translate into practice, and even a contested approach to what it means to hold power and be accountable for its exercise. In short, management theory and good social work practice need not be in opposition. On the contrary, both should be informed by a common understanding of individual and group behaviour. Indeed, the purpose of good management is not self-perpetuation or tyrannical dictatorship but to deliver the vision and objectives of the organisation.

The real challenge for social work managers is not to emulate the more negative and perhaps distorted stereotypes of the private business world in seeing who can run the leanest and fittest organisation, the 'tightest ship', the 'biggest empire', or who can hire and fire with the greatest abandon. Rather, it is to absorb those ideas emerging from the business world which suggest that success lies in valuing, fostering and listening to the workforce, hearing and responding to the 'customer', managing diversity not conformity and seeking to build in flexibility at every stage. It is perfectly possible for a manager who is a 'people person' to build their own style around this, and for that style to be one that empowers others to give of their best, not to fit in with narrow diktats from above. The advent of computers in social work offices, for example, has made workers feel that they are filling in little boxes on the screen and being boxed in themselves in the process. Yet the lightning speed and infinite networks of the computer age could equally well be used to open up communication – to send ideas, insights and concerns speeding round the organisation to where they can be used in planning and improving services, and to draw in information from the internet so that policy and practice can be grounded in research-generated knowledge. It is frankly ridiculous to use such boundary-breaking technology only for recording and monitoring systems that make people feel like the lowliest penpushers of the Victorian era.

Similarly, the imposition of uniform standards into service aims and contracting, instead of being a levelling down to spread resources as thinly as possible, could be a levelling up to spread the principles of equality and social justice – because these do not always cost more but they do require more rigorous implementation. There is no reason why computerised case recording could not be used to make a note of every service user's first language and ensure that interpreter services were prebooked for each interview. There is no reason why women using every kind of service right across a local authority could not automatically be asked (in a safe and confidential way) whether they are experiencing domestic violence or why the resultant statistics could not be used to establish an authority-wide policy and practice response. Nor is there any obstacle to collating information on the internal operation of disability legislation so as to make planned changes to working practices and workplace design, as opposed to incremental adaptations as the need arises.

In other words, when the principles of anti-oppressive practice are translated into anti-oppressive policy, they open up exciting new horizons for managers that could begin to make a reality of the rhetoric of social inclusion. Surely there can be no better reason to aspire to be a manager than to want to make one's mark in this kind of way?

And the world moves on

It actually felt outdated still to be writing in Chapter 7 about the oppression of particular social groups as needing attention in social work organisations. We have known for many years what we ought to be doing and there is little excuse for the slow rate of progress. Social work is being outstripped in many commercial contexts (here and overseas) in provision for women returners, black managers, disabled employees, gay and lesbian staff and so on. We talk the talk better than we walk the walk in many respects.

Meanwhile, cutting-edge management theory has moved on to issues of social justice and human rights at a global and environmental level. From corporate social responsibility audits of businesses to sustainable development in education, interest in the ethical stance leaders take has marked a shift towards 'values aware' management. There is an international environmental standard, ISO 14001, that both public and private sector bodies are achieving for reasons of efficiency, cost and reputation, as well as social conscience. Many individuals now choose, similarly, to invest in savings that avoid socially and environmentally harmful products such as the arms trade and the tobacco industry.

Because the 'consumers' of social work typically do not have many choices about what services they receive, they are unlikely to boycott meals on wheels, just because they are delivered in a petrol-hungry van, or to question whether the county council has its capital ethically invested. They do, however, expect the standards of central and local government, and charitable organisations, to be transparently honest and based on 'ordinary common decency', not only in dealing with service users and staff, but also in pursuing the wider responsibilities of 'corporate citizenship' in the local community (Pettinger, 1997, pp. 156–7). And it is also true that, these days, the threat of global economic meltdown or planetary climate change seems almost as likely to block the nation's ability to provide adequate welfare coverage in the future as do more localised considerations. Consequently, the manager of tomorrow may need to be able to see everything connecting to everything else on a scope that the systems theorists never dreamt of. Organisational Gaia, perhaps.

Today's generation of social work students take an active interest in such widespread issues and, if the incumbent generation does not stifle their initiative and energies, they are well placed to make a difference in the future. The study of management and organisational theory need not be about how to wear a suit and talk in statistics. It can be about how to work together, learn together and survive together in a world where every assumption has been turned upside down, where the only certainty is uncertainty, and where the most valued skill may be the ability to think on the broadest canvas, with the most variables in play, and the greatest respect for all the people whose well-being is at risk.

This is where principles and skills come together, in a way that confirms good social work as lying at the heart of good management. Every social worker has a part to play in management, and every manager, social work qualified or not, has a lot to learn from social work.

References

Adams, R. (1998) *Quality Social Work*, Basingstoke: Macmillan.

Aldridge, M. (1996) 'Dragged to market: being a profession in the postmodern world', *British Journal of Social Work*, 26(2), pp. 177–94.

Allan, M., Bhavnani, R. and French, K. (for the DoH/SSI) (1992) *Promoting Women: Management Development and Training for Women in Social Services Departments*, London: HMSO.

Anderson, C. R. (1985) *Management: Skills, Function and Organisation Performance*, Dubuque, IO: Brown.

Andrew, F. (1996) *Not Just Black and White: An Exploration of Opportunities and Barriers to the Development of Black Managers in Public Services*, London: Office for Public Management.

Argyris, C. (1957) *Personality and Organization*, New York: Harper.

Argyris, C. and Schön, D. A. (1978) *Organizational Learning: A Theory of Action Perspective*, Reading, MA: Addison-Wesley.

Atherton, J. S. (1986) *Professional Supervision in Group Care: A Contract-Based Approach*, London: Tavistock.

Audit Commission (1995) *On Merit: Recruitment in Local Government*, London: HMSO.

Balloch, S. and Taylor, M. (eds) (2001) *Partnership Working: Policy and Practice*, Bristol: Policy Press.

Balloch, S., Pahl, J. and McLean, J. (1998) 'Working in the social services: job satisfaction, stress and violence', *British Journal of Social Work*, 28, pp. 329–50.

Balloch, S., Andrew, T., Ginn, J., McLean, J., Pahl, J. and Williams, J. (1995) *Working in the Social Services*, London: National Institute for Social Work.

Bamford, T. (1982) *Managing Social Work*, London: Tavistock.

Barter, S. (1997) 'Social work students with personal experience of sexual abuse: implications for Diploma in Social Work programme providers', *Social Work Education*, 16(2), pp. 113–32.

Bensted, J., Brown, A., Forbes, C. and Wall, R. (1994) 'Men working with men in groups: masculinity and crime', *Groupwork*, 7(1), pp. 37–49.

Bhatti-Sinclair, K. (1996) *Developing Black Mentors and Consultants Schemes in Social Work Education: A Guidance Handbook for Black and Minority Ethnic Students, Practice Teachers, Tutors and Programme Providers*, Southampton: University of Southampton, Department of Social Work Studies.

Bilson, A. and Ross, S. (1999) *Social Work Management and Practice: Systems Principles*, 2nd edn, London: Jessica Kingsley.

Blair, T. (2001) Speech by the Prime Minister, 'Reform of public services', 16 July. http://www.number-10.gov.uk/output/Page1594.asp.

Bond, H. (1996) 'Tell it like it is', *Community Care*, 2–8 May, p. 10.

Bowen, W. G. and Bok, D. (1998) *The Shape of the River: Long-Term Consequences of Considering Race in College and University Admissions*, Princeton, NJ: Princeton University Press.

Brown, A. (1992) *Groupwork*, 3rd edn, Aldershot: Ashgate.

Brown, A. and Bourne, I. (1996) *The Social Work Supervisor: Supervision in Community, Day Care and Residential Settings*, Buckingham: Open University Press.

Bunning, R. L. (1979) 'The Delphi technique: a projection tool for serious enquiry', in Jones, J. E. and Pfeiffer, J. W. (eds) *Annual Handbook for Group Facilitators*, La Jolla, CA: University Associates, pp. 174–81.

Burstow, B. (1992) *Feminist Therapy: Working in the Context of Violence*, Newbury Park, CA: Sage.

Burton, J. (1998) *Managing Residential Care*, London: Routledge.

Butt, J. and Mirza, K. (1996) *Social Care and Black Communities: A Review of Recent Research Studies*, London: HMSO.

Carnall, C. (1995) *Managing Change in Organizations*, 2nd edn, London: Prentice Hall International.

Carter Hood, P., Everitt, A. and Runnicles, D. (1998) 'Femininity, sexuality and professionalism in the children's departments', *British Journal of Social Work*, 28, pp. 471–90.

Casson, S. F and Manning, B. (1997) *Total Quality in Child Protection: A Manager's Guide*, Lyme Regis: Russell House Publishing.

CCETSW (Central Council for Education and Training in Social Work) (1997) *Assuring Quality for Post Qualifying Education and Training – 1. Requirements for the Post Qualifying and Advanced Awards in Social Work*, London: CCETSW.

Chetkow-Yanoov, B. (1992) *Social Work Practice: A Systems Approach*, Binghamton, NY: Haworth.

Clarke, J. and Newman, J. (1997) *The Managerial State: Power, Politics and Ideology in the Remaking of Social Welfare*, London: Sage.

Clegg, S. R. (1990) *Modern Organizations: Organization Studies in the Postmodern World*, London: Sage.

Clutterbuck, D. and Crainer, S. (1990) *Makers of Management: Men and Women who Changed the Business World,* London: Guild Publishing.

Cockburn, C. (1991) *In the Way of Women: Men's Resistance to Sex Equality in Organizations,* Basingstoke: Macmillan – now Palgrave Macmillan.

Cohen, S. (1975) 'It's all right for you to talk: political and sociological manifestos for social action', in Bailey, R. and Brake, M. (eds) *Radical Social Work,* London: Edward Arnold.

Coleman, G. (1991) *Investigating Organisations: A Feminist Approach,* Bristol: University of Bristol, School for Advanced Urban Studies.

Collinge, M., Blakey, C. and Jones, D. N. (1986) 'The one way screen', *Community Care,* 25 September, pp. 16–17.

Collinson, D. L. and Hearn, J. (1996) *Men as Managers, Managers as Men,* London: Sage.

Colton, M. and Vanstone, M. (1998) 'Sexual abuse by men who work with children: an exploratory study', *British Journal of Social Work,* 28(4), pp. 511–23.

CRE (Commission for Racial Equality) (1993) *Towards Fair Selection,* London: Commission for Racial Equality.

CRE (Commission for Racial Equality) (1996) 'Twenty years of action for equality', *CRE-Connections: Bulletin of Racial Equality,* 7, June, p. 1.

CRE (Commission for Racial Equality) (1997) '1997: Countdown to the millennium on racial equality', *News Release,* 629, London: CRE.

Cosis Brown, H. (1998) *Social Work and Sexuality: Working with Lesbians and Gay Men,* Basingstoke: Macmillan – now Palgrave Macmillan.

Coulshed, V and Orme, J. (1998) *Social Work Practice: An Introduction,* Basingstoke: Macmillan – now Palgrave Macmillan.

Coyle, A. (1989) 'Women in management: a suitable case for treatment?', *Feminist Review,* 31, pp. 117–25.

Dadswell, T. (1999) 'Under suspicion', *Professional Social Work,* February, pp. 6–7.

Daly, N. (1998) 'Care or scare?', *Community Care,* 30 July–5 August, p. 19.

Darvill, G. (1998a) 'Making the move into management', *Professional Social Work,* October, p. 14.

Darvill, G. (1998b) *Organisation, People and Standards. Use of Formal Standards in Social Services: Report of a Survey (ADSS and NISW),* London: National Institute for Social Work.

Davies, D. and Neal, C. (eds) (1996) *Pink Therapy: A Guide for Counsellors and Therapists Working with Lesbian, Gay and Bisexual Clients,* Buckingham: Open University Press.

DETR (Department of the Environment, Transport and the Regions) (1998) *Modernising Local Government: Improving Local Services through Best Value,* London: Stationery Office.

DoH (Department of Health) (1998a) *Modernising Social Services: Promoting Independence, Improving Protection, Raising Standards,* London: Stationery Office.

DoH (Department of Health) (1998b) *The Quality Protects Programme: Transforming Children's Services,* London: Department of Health, LAC(98)28.

DoH (Department of Health) (1999) *The Government's Objectives for Children's Social Services,* London: Department of Health.

DoH/SSI (Department of Health Social Services Inspectorate) and the Audit Commission (2002) *Tracking the Changes: Joint Review Team Sixth Annual Report, 2001/02,* London: Audit Commission.

DoH/SSI (Department of Health Social Services Inspectorate) and the Audit Commission (2003) *A Report of the Joint Review of Social Services in Kirklees Metropolitan Council,* London: Audit Commission.

DoH/SSI (Department of Health Social Services Inspectorate) and the Scottish Office Social Work Services Group (1991) *Care Management and Assessment: Practitioners' Guide,* London: HMSO.

Dessler, G. (1985) *Management Fundamentals,* Reston, VA: Reston.

Dominelli, L. (1997) *Anti-Racist Social Work: A Challenge for White Practitioners and Educators,* 2nd edn, Basingstoke: Macmillan – now Palgrave Macmillan.

Dominelli, L. and McLeod, E. (1989) *Feminist Social Work,* Basingstoke: Macmillan – now Palgrave Macmillan.

Drucker, P. F. (1954) *The Practice of Management,* New York: Harper & Row.

Drucker, P. F. (1977) *Management,* London: Pan.

Dunnachie, H. (1992) 'Approaches to quality systems', in Kelly, D. and Warr, B. (eds) *Quality Counts: Achieving Quality in Social Care Services,* London: Whiting & Birch.

Ellis, R. and Whittington, D. (1998) *Quality Assurance in Social Care: An Introductory Workbook,* London: Arnold.

EOC (Equal Opportunities Commission) for Northern Ireland (1998) *What Price Sex Equality: Making a Sex Discrimination Complaint,* Belfast: Equal Opportunities Commission for Northern Ireland.

Eraut, M. (1994) *Developing Professional Knowledge and Competence,* London: Falmer.

Fisher, R. and Ury, W. (1983) *Getting to Yes,* New York: Penguin.

Follett, M. P. (1925) 'Constructive conflict', paper presented to a Bureau of Personnel Administration conference group, New York, January

1925, reproduced in Metcalf, H. C. and Urwick, L. (eds) *Dynamic Admnistration: The Collected Papers of Mary Parker Follett*, London: Sir Isaac Pitman and Sons Ltd.

Ford, D. L. and Nemiroff, P. M. (1975) 'Applied group problem-solving: the nominal group technique', in *Annual Handbook for Group Facilitators*, La Jolla, CA: University Associates, pp. 179–82.

Ford, K. and Jones, A. (1987) *Student Supervision,* London: Macmillan – now Palgrave Macmillan.

Foster, G. (1996) *Getting What You Want: A Short Guide to Career Development for Senior Women Managers,* London: National Institute for Social Work.

Foster, G. and Phillipson, J. (1994) *Making Positive Choices. Career Development for Women in Social Care: What Women Can Do,* London: National Institute for Social Work.

Foster, J. (1997) A woman's liberation', *Community Care,* 4–10 December, pp. 18–19.

Franks, S. (1999) *Having None of It: Women, Men and the Future of Work,* London: Granta.

French, J. R. P. and Raven, B. (1959) 'The bases of social power', in Cartwright, D. (ed.) *Studies in Social Power,* Ann Arbor: University of Michigan.

Friedman, R., Kane, M. and Cornfield, D. B. (1998) 'Social support and career optimism: examining the effectiveness of network groups among black managers', *Human Relations,* 51(9), pp. 1155–77.

Galligan, D. (1992) 'Procedural rights and social welfare', in Coote, A. (ed.) *The Welfare of Citizens,* London: Rivers Oram Press.

Gann, N. (1996) *Managing Change in Voluntary Organizations: A Guide to Practice,* Buckingham: Open University Press.

Garrett, P. M. (1999) 'Mapping child-care social work in the final years of the twentieth century: a critical response to the "looking after children" system', *British Journal of Social Work,* 29(1), pp. 27–47.

Gensen, J. (1996) *Men as Workers in Childcare Services,* Brussels: European Commission.

Geus, A. de (1997) *The Living Company,* Boston, MA: Harvard Business School Press.

Goleman, D. (1996) *Emotional Intelligence: Why It Can Matter More Than IQ,* London: Bloomsbury.

Grover, R. (1992) 'Rest assured', *Community Care,* 3 December, p. 16.

Handy, C. (1993) *Understanding Organizations,* 4th edn, Harmondsworth: Penguin.

Handy, C. (1995) *The Age of Unreason,* 3rd edn, London: Arrow.

Hardman, K. (1997) 'Social workers' attitudes to lesbian clients', *The British Journal of Social Work,* 27(4), pp. 545–63.

Haynes, P. (2003) *Managing Complexity in the Public Services*, Maidenhead: Open University Press.

Hearn, J. and Parkin, W. (1995) *Sex at Work: The Power and Paradox of Organisation Sexuality*, rev. edn, London: Prentice Hall/Harvester Wheatsheaf.

Hersey, P. and Blanchard, K. H. (1982) *Management of Organisational Behavior: Utilising Human Resources*, Englewood Cliffs, NJ: Prentice Hall.

Hibbert, P. (2003) *Voices and Choices: Young People Participating in Inspections. Learning from the Listening and Responding Component of Social Services Inspectorate Inspections of Local Authority Children's Services*, London: Barnardo's.

Hill, M. (1997) *The Policy Process in the Modern State*, 3rd edn, London: Prentice Hall.

Hirst, J. (1998) 'Caught in the spotlight', *Community Care*, 23–29 July, p. 89.

Hofstede G. (1980) *Culture's Consequences*, Newbury Park, CA: Sage.

Home, A. (1993) 'The juggling act: the multiple role woman in social work education', *Canadian Social Work Review*, 10(2), pp. 141–56.

Horwath, J. (1996) 'Undertaking a training needs analysis within a social care organisation', in Connelly, N. (ed.) *Training Social Services Staff: Evidence from New Research*, London: National Institute for Social Work, Research in Social Work Education, 4.

Horwath, J. and Morrison, T. (1999) *Effective Staff Training in Social Care*, London: Routledge.

Hughes, W. H. (1986) *Report of the Inquiry into Children's Homes and Hostels*, Belfast: HMSO.

Hunt, G. (ed.) (1998) *Whistleblowing in the Social Services: Public Accountability and Professional Practice*, London: Arnold.

Hunter, M. (1999) 'A third way for charities?', *Community Care*, 7–13 January, pp. 18–19.

Hunter, T. and Blackmore, J. (2003) 'Hunter-gatherer or farmer?', *Care and Health*, 49, pp. 19–21.

Itzin, C. (1995) 'Crafting strategy to create women-friendly work', in Itzin, C. and Newman, J. (eds) *Gender, Culture and Organizational Change: Putting Theory into Practice*, London: Routledge.

Ixer, G. (1999) 'There's no such thing as reflection', *British Journal of Social Work*, 29(4), pp. 513–27.

Jackson, A. C. and Donovan, F. H. (1999) *Managing to Survive: Managerial Practice in Not-for-Profit Organizations*, Buckingham: Open University Press.

Janis, I. L. (1971) 'Groupthink', *Psychology Today*, 5(6), pp. 43–6.

Johnstone, H. (1995) 'Beat the interview blues', *London Evening Standard*, Business recruitment feature, 8 March, p. 46.

JICC (Joint Initiative for Community Care) (1998) *Training for the Caring Business: A Manager's Guide*, 2nd edn, Milton Keynes: JICC.

Joint Reviews (2004) *Old Virtues, New Virtues: an Overview of the Changes in Social Care Services Over the Seven Years of Joint Reviews in England 1996–2003*, London: Audit Commission.

Jones, A. (1996) *Report of the Examination Team on Child Care and Practice in North Wales*, London: HMSO.

Jones, A., Phillips,. M. and Maynard, C. (1992) *A Home from Home: The Experience of Black Residential Projects as a Focus of Good Practice*, London: National Institute for Social Work.

Jones, D. (1999a) 'Frameworks for action', *Professional Social Work*, December, pp. 16–17.

Jones, D. (1999b) 'Regulating social work: key questions', *Practice*, 11(3), pp. 55–63.

Jones, D. (1999c) 'Surviving joint reviews', *Professional Social Work*, August, p. 17.

Jones, D. N. (2000) *People Need People: Releasing the Potential of People Working in Social Services*, London: Audit Commission, Department of Health and Office of the National Assembly for Wales.

Kahan, B. (1994) *Growing up in Groups*, London: National Institute for Social Work Research.

Kanter, R. M. (1989) *When Giants Learn to Dance: Mastering the Challenges of Strategy, Management, and Careers in the 1990s*, London: Simon & Schuster.

Kanter, R. M. (1991) 'Change-master skills: what it takes to be creative', in Henry, J. and Walker, D. (eds) *Managing Innovation*, London: Sage.

Kara, H. and Muir, P. (2003) *Commissioning Consultancy: Managing Outside Expertise to Improve Your Services*, Lyme Regis: Russell House Publishing.

Kearney, P. (1999) *Managing Practice: Report on the Management of Practice Expertise Project*, London: National Institute for Social Work.

Kendall, J. with Almond, S. (1998) *The UK Voluntary (Third) Sector in Comparative Perspective: Exceptional Growth and Transformation*, Canterbury: Personal Social Services Research Unit.

Kendrick, A. (1997) *Safeguarding Children Living Away from Home from Abuse: A Literature Review*, in Kent, R. (ed.) *Children's Safeguards Review*, Edinburgh: Stationery Office.

Kent, R. (ed.) (1997) *Children's Safeguards Review*, Edinburgh: Stationery Office.

Knapham, J. and Morrison, T. (1998) *Making the Most of Supervision in Health and Social Care: A Self Development Manual for Supervisees*, Brighton: Pavilion Publishing.

Kotter, J. and Schlesinger, L. (1979) 'Choosing strategies for change', *Harvard Business Review*, March–April, pp. 106–14.

Lance, H. and Bunch, C. (1998) *Choices for Change: A Guide to Training and Development Opportunities for Women Managers in the Personal Social Services*, London: The Learning Agency.

Lawler, J. and Hearn, J. (1997) 'The managers of social work: the experiences and identifications of third tier social services managers and the implications for future practice', *British Journal of Social Work*, 27(2), pp. 191–218.

Leigh, A. (1983) *Decisions, Decisions! A Practical Management Guide to Problem-Solving and Decision-Making*, Aldershot: Gower.

Leigh, A. (1988) *Effective Change: Twenty Ways to Make it Happen*, London: Institute of Personnel Management.

Levy, A. and Kahan, B. (1991) *The Pindown Experience and the Protection of Children: The Report for the Staffordshire Child Care Inquiry*, Stafford: Staffordshire County Council.

Lewin, K. (1951) *Field Theory in Social Science*, New York: Harper & Row.

Likert, R. (1961) *New Patterns of Management*, New York: McGraw-Hill.

Lipsky, M. (1980) *Street-Level Bureaucracy: Dilemmas of the Individual in Public Services*, New York: Russell Sage Foundation.

Lishman, J. (1998) 'Personal and professional development', in Adams, R., Dominelli, L. and Payne, M. (eds) *Social Work: Themes, Issues and Critical Debates*, Basingstoke: Macmillan – now Palgrave Macmillan.

LGMB (Local Government Management Board) and the ADSS (Association of Directors of Social Services) (1993) *Social Services Workforce Analysis: 1992 Survey. Main Report*, London: LGMB.

Logan, J., Kershaw, S., Karban, K., Mills, S., Trotter, J. and Sinclair, M. (1996) *Confronting Prejudice: Lesbian and Gay Issues in Social Work Education*, Aldershot: Arena.

Luciano, P. R. (1979) 'The systems view of organisations: dynamics of organisational change', in *Annual Handbook for Group Facilitators*, La Jolla, CA: University Associates.

Machiavelli, N. (1961) *The Prince*, Harmondsworth: Penguin (originally written in 1541).

Maddock, S. (1999) *Challenging Women*, London: Sage.

Maslow, A. H. (1954) *Motivation and Personality*, New York: Harper & Row.

Maxwell, R. J. (1984) 'Quality assessment in health: perspectives in NHS management', *British Medical Journal*, 288, pp. 1470–2.

McFarlane, L. (1998) *Diagnosis Homophobic: The Experiences of Lesbians, Gay Men and Bisexuals in Mental Health Services*, 34 Hartham Road, London N7 9JL: Project for Advice, Counselling and Education (PACE).

McGregor, D. (1960) *The Human Side of Enterprise*, Sydney: McGraw-Hill Australia.

McKay, R. (1999) 'Scots open new umbrella group for ethnic minorities', *Community Care*, 4–10 November, p. 11.

McKay, R. (2002) 'New managers feel unprepared for role', *Community Care*, 5–11 September, p. 14.

McKenna, E. and Beech, N. (1995) *The Essence of Human Resource Management*, Hemel Hempstead: Prentice Hall Europe.

Minister for Disabled People (1996a) *The Disability Discrimination Act 1995: Are You Facing Employment Discrimination?*, DL180.

Minister for Disabled People (1996b) *The Disability Discrimination Act 1995: A Guide for Everybody*, DL160.

Mintzberg, H. (1973) *The Nature of Managerial Work*, New York: Harper & Row.

Mintzberg, H. (1989) 'The structuring of organizations', in Asch, D. and Bowman, C. (eds) *Readings in Strategic Management*, London: Macmillan – now Palgrave Macmillan.

Moore, J. I. (1992) *Writers on Strategy and Strategic Management: The Theory of Strategy and the Practice of Strategic Management at Enterprise, Corporate, Business and Functional Levels*, Harmondsworth: Penguin.

Morgan, C. and Murgatroyd, S. J. (1994) *Total Quality Management in the Public Sector*, Buckingham: Open University Press.

Morgan, G. (1986) *Images of Organization*, Thousand Oaks, CA: Sage.

Morgan, G. (1993) *Imaginization: the Art of Creative Management*, Newbury Park, CA: Sage.

Mullender, A. (1996) *Rethinking Domestic Violence: The Social Work and Probation Response*, London: Routledge.

Mullender, A. (ed.) (1999) *We Are Family: Sibling Relationships in Placement and Beyond*, London: British Agencies for Adoption and Fostering.

Murray, C. (1997) 'Gender inequality in social work management: cause for pessimism or signs of progress?', in Keeble, L. and Fisher, M. (eds) *Making a Difference: Women and Career Progression in Social Services. Report of a National Seminar at the Social Work Research Centre, University of Stirling*, London: National Institute for Social Work.

NISW (1995) *Managing Information and Change*, London: National Institute for Social Work, *Policy Briefings*, 11.

NISW (1996) *The Social Services Information Agenda*, London: National Institute for Social Work, *NISW Briefing*, 17.

NISW (1998) *The Social Services Workforce Studies: Summary*, London: National Institute for Social Work.

NISW (1999) *Violence Against Social Care Workers*, London: National Institute for Social Work, *NISW Briefing*, 26.

NISW (2001) *Special Measures Interventions: Working in Local Authorities to Improve Performance in Social Services*, London: National Institute for Social Work, *NISW Briefing*, 32.

Nottage, A. (for the DoH/SSI) (1991) *Women in Social Services: A Neglected Resource*, London: HMSO.

Nuffield Institute for Health/United Kingdom Homecare Association (1997) *What Do Users and Carers Want from Domiciliary Care?*, Leeds: Nuffield Institute for Health, Community Care Division.

ODPM (Office of the Deputy Prime Minister) (2001) *Strong Local Leadership: Quality Public Services*, London: Stationery Office.

Office for Public Management (1995) *Setting the Agenda: Black Managers in Public Services. A Conference Held in September 1994 by the Office for Public Management*, London: Office for Public Management.

Oliver, M. and Barnes, C. (1998) *Disabled People and Social Policy: From Exclusion to Inclusion*, Harlow: Longman.

Parkin, D. and Maddock, S. (1995) 'A gender typology of organizational culture', in Itzin, C. and Newman, J. (eds) *Gender, Culture and Organizational Change: Putting Theory into Practice*, London: Routledge.

Paterson, J. (1999) *Disability Rights Handbook: April 1999–April 2000*, 24th edn, London: Disability Alliance Educational and Research Association.

Payne, M. (2000) *Teamwork in Multiprofessional Care*, Basingstoke: Palgrave – now Palgrave Macmillan.

Pernell, R. B. (1986) 'Empowerment and social group work', in Parries, M. (ed.) *Innovations in Social Group Work: Feedback from Practice to Theory*, Binghamton, NY: Haworth.

Peter, L. J. (1970) *The Peter Principle*, Harmondsworth: Penguin.

Peters, T. J. (1988) *Thriving on Chaos: Handbook for a Management Revolution*, London: Macmillan – now Palgrave Macmillan.

Peters, T. J. and Waterman, R. H. (1982) *In Search of Excellence: Lessons from America's Best-Run Companies*, New York: Warner Books/London: Harper & Row.

Pettinger, R. (1997) *Introduction to Management*, 2nd edn, Basingstoke: Macmillan – now Palgrave Macmillan.

Pfeffer, N. and Coote, A. (1991) *Is Quality Good for You? A Critical Review of Quality Assurance in Welfare Services*, London: Institute of Public Policy Research, Paper 5.

Pharr, S. (1988) *Homophobia: A Weapon of Sexism,* Little Rock, AR: Chardon Press.

Piggott, J. B. and Piggott, G. (1992) 'Total quality management (TQM): the way ahead', in Kelly, D. and Wan, B. (eds) *Quality Counts: Achieving Quality in Social Care Services,* London: Whiting & Birch.

Pottage, D. and Evans, M. (1992) *Workbased Stress: Prescription is Not the Cure,* London: National Institute for Social Work, *Discussion Paper,* 1.

Pottage, D. and Evans, M. (1994) *The Competent Workplace: The View from Within,* London: National Institute for Social Work, *Discussion Paper,* 2.

Priestley, M. (1998) 'Discourse and resistance in care assessment: integrated living and community care', *British Journal of Social Work,* 28(5), pp. 659–73.

Pringle, K. (1992/3) 'Child sexual abuse perpetrated by welfare personnel and the problem of men', *Critical Social Policy,* Issue 36, 12(3), pp. 4–19.

Pugh, D. (1993) 'Understanding and managing organizational change', in Mabey, C. and Mayon-White, B. (eds) *Managing Change,* 2nd edn, London: Paul Chapman.

Qureshi, H. (1998) 'Outcomes and local authorities', in Balloch, S. (ed.) *Outcomes of Social Care: A Question of Quality?,* London: National Institute for Social Work, Social Services Policy Forum, Paper 6.

Rosen, G. (ed.) (1999) *Managing Team Development: A Short Guide for Teams and Team Managers,* London: National Institute for Social Work.

Salaman, G. (1992) *Human Resource Strategies,* London: Sage.

Sanderson, T. (1993) *Assertively Gay: How to Build Gay Self-Esteem,* London: The Other Way Press.

Sapey, B. (1997) 'Social work tomorrow: towards a critical understanding of technology in social work', *British Journal of Social Work,* 27(6), pp. 803–14.

Schein, E. H. (1985) *Organizational Culture and Leadership,* San Francisco: Jossey Bass.

Schön, D. A. (1983) *The Reflective Practitioner,* New York: Basic Books.

Schwehr, B. (1999) 'Caring about stress', *Community Care,* 5–11 August, p. 27.

Scottish Office (1998) *The Scottish Office Response to the Children's Safeguards Review,* Edinburgh: Scottish Office.

Seebohm Report (1968) *Report of the Committee on Local Authority and Allied Personal Social Services,* Cmnd 3703, London: HMSO.

Senge, P. M. (1992) *The Fifth Discipline: The Art and Practice of the Learning Organization,* London: Century Business.

Shepherd, C. (1997) 'Research update note on ME/CFS', *British Journal of Social Work*, 27(5), pp. 755–60.

Skellington, R. with Morris, P. (1992) *'Race' in Britain Today*, London: Sage.

Skinner, A. (1992) *Another Kind of Home: A Review of Residential Child Care*, Edinburgh: HMSO.

Smale, G. (1996) *Mapping Change and Innovation*, London: NISW.

Smale, G. (1997) *Managing Change through Innovation*, London: NISW.

Smith, J. (1999) 'Prior criminality and employment of social workers with substantial access to children: a decision board analysis', *British Journal of Social Work*, 29(1), pp. 49–68.

Spender, D. (1990) *Man Made Language*, London: Pandora.

Stacey, R. D. (2000) *Strategic Management and Organisational Dynamics: The Challenge of Complexity*, 3rd edn, Harlow: Pearson Education.

Steele, J. (1999) *Wasted Values: Harnessing the Commitment of Public Managers*, London: Public Management Foundation.

Stock Whitaker, D. (1975) 'Some conditions for effective work with groups', *British Journal of Social Work*, 5(4), pp. 423–39.

Stubbs, P. (1985) 'The employment of black social workers: from "ethnic sensitivity" to anti-racism', *Critical Social Policy*, 12, pp. 6–27.

Support Force for Children's Residential Care (1995) *Code of Practice for the Employment of Residential Child Care Workers*, London: Department of Health.

Tannen, D. (1995) *Talking from 9 to 5: How Women's and Men's Conversational Styles Affect Who Gets Heard, Who Gets Credit and What Gets Done at Work*, London: Virago (also available in paperback, published in 1996, as *Talking from 9 to 5: Women and Men at Work – Language, Sex and Power*, London: Virago).

Tannenbaum, R. and Schmidt, W. (1973) 'How to choose a leadership pattern', *Harvard Business Review*, May–June.

Tanton, M. (1994) *Women in Management: A Developing Presence*, London: Routledge.

Thompson, A. (1999) 'Shaping up for the future', *Community Care*, 25–31 March, pp. 22–3.

Thompson, N. (2002a) *People Skills*, 2nd edn, Basingstoke: Palgrave Macmillan.

Thompson, N. (2002b) 'Research into practice', *Community Care*, 19–25 September, p. 52.

Thompson, N. (2003) *Promoting Equality: Challenging Discrimination and Oppression in the Human Services*, 2nd edn, Basingstoke: Palgrave Macmillan.

Thompson, N., Stradling, S. and Murphy, M. (1994) *Dealing with Stress*, Basingstoke: Macmillan – now Palgrave Macmillan.

Thompson, N., Stradling, S., Murphy, M. and O'Neill, P. (1996) 'Stress and organizational culture', *British Journal of Social Work,* 26, pp. 647–66.

Torrington, D. and Hall, L. (1998) *Human Resource Management,* 4th edn, Hemel Hempstead: Prentice Hall Europe.

Townley, B. (1994) *Retraining Human Resource Management: Power Ethics and the Subject at Work,* London: Sage.

Turner, M. (1995) 'Supervising', in Carter, P., Jeffs, T. and Smith, M. K. (eds) *Social Working,* Basingstoke: Macmillan – now Palgrave Macmillan.

Utting, W. (1987) *People Like Us: The Report of the Review of Safeguards for Children Living Away from Home,* London: Stationery Office.

Utting, W (1997) *Children in Public Care: A Review of Residential Child Care,* London: HMSO.

Wallis, L. and Frost, N. (1998) *Cause for Complaint,* London: Children's Society.

Walsh, K. (1995) 'Quality through markets: the new public service management', in Wilkinson, A. and Willmott, H. (eds) *Making Quality Critical: New Perspectives on Organizational Change,* London: Routledge.

Warham, J. (1975) *An Introduction to Administration for Social Workers,* London: Routledge & Kegan Paul.

Warner, N. (1992) *Choosing with Care: The Report of the Committee of Inquiry into the Selection, Development and Management of Staff in Children's Homes,* London: HMSO.

Warr, B. and Kelly, D. (1992) 'What is meant by quality in social care', in Kelly, D. and Warr, B. (eds) *Quality Counts: Achieving Quality in Social Care Services,* London: Whiting & Birch.

Weber, M. (1947) *The Theory of Social and Economic Organization,* New York: Free Press.

Weiner, M. E. (1982) *Human Services Management: Analysis and Applications,* Itasca, IL: Dorsey.

Westley, F. and Mintzberg, H. (1991) 'Visionary leadership and strategic management', in Henry, J. and Walker, D. (eds) *Managing Innovation,* London: Sage.

Williams, G. and McCreadie, J. (1982) *Ty Mawr Community Homes Inquiry,* Cwmbran: Gwent County Council.

Wilson, F. M. (2003) *Organizational Behaviour and Gender,* 2nd edn, Aldershot: Ashgate.

Zander, B. and Zander, R. S. (2000) *The Art of Possibility,* Boston, MA: Harvard Business School Press.

Index